Clinical Care

T0258724

Nursing in General Practice: Clinical Care

JOINT EDITORS

BARBARA STILWELL
Primary Health Care Researcher,
West Lambeth Health Authority

and

RICHARD HOBBS
Senior Lecturer, Department of General Practice
University of Birmingham

RADCLIFFE MEDICAL PRESS
OXFORD

British Library Cataloguing in Publication Data

Stilwell, Barbara
  Nursing in general practice: clinical care
  I. Title   II. Hobbs, Richard
  610.73

  ISBN 1 870905 46 6

Printed and bound in Great Britain
by Billing & Sons Limited, Worcester.
Typeset by Advance Typesetting, Oxfordshire

Contents

Foreword   vii

List of Authors   ix

Preface   xi

1. The Developing Role of the Practice Nurse in   1
       Great Britain
    Richard Hobbs and Barbara Stilwell

2. General Practice and the Primary Care Team   11
    Richard Hobbs

3. Communication Skills   27
    Barbara Stilwell and Peter Havelock

4. Health Education and the Oxford Prevention of   47
       Heart Attack and Stroke Project
    Elaine Fullard, with a contribution by Elizabeth Armstrong

5. Care of Patients with Asthma   65
    Greta Barnes

6. Care of Patients with Hypertension   91
    Theo Schofield and Lilian Vincent

7. Care of Patients with Diabetes Mellitus   113
    Richard Hobbs and Ellen Murray

8. First Aid and Emergencies   149
    Phyllis Moore

9   The Way Forward   167
    Barbara Stilwell and Richard Hobbs

Index   171

Foreword

THE speed of change in medicine has dramatically accelerated during the last half of this century posing new problems for all concerned with care. There are at least four major factors behind this and they include firstly the fact that hospital based medical care has become more technical, more specialized and much more expensive. Next, there have been major changes in the demography of the population and in disease patterns to accompany this. The population is growing older and infectious diseases occupy a less prominent position so we are all more concerned with degenerative disease and patients with multiple problems. Then, our concern with ecological issues and the environment has meant that health promotion and disease prevention are now of major concern to many people and, lastly, there has been a general rise in standards of living for most people making us more mobile. There are, of course, other factors such as those associated with urban or inner city dwelling, but these have meant that the pressures for treating people outside hospital are great. These pressures are both social and clinical, as well as purely economic.

General practice is having to become increasingly sophisticated and it is apparent that even the better organized doctors cannot cope alone with the volume of work. They have not the time, but more importantly there are skills, attitudes and knowledge needed that they do not possess either. Hence the dramatic rise in numbers of practice nurses within the past ten years.

It would be foolish to believe that we have yet worked out completely how doctors and nurses are to work together in this new arena. What are the boundaries of each other's work? What training and monitoring of skill is required? How do we work together so that some of the tensions that exist between the two professions in other fields are minimized? What we do have now is growing evidence that where we do work together, patient care is greatly enhanced.

So far the areas in which this has been best tested have been in chronic disease—asthma, diabetes and hypertension; in preventive care to the middle-aged, and in treatment room procedures. This volume deals with these matters. There are other areas where it seems such shared care has much to offer. They include comprehensive health education and health promotion, problems of women, minor anxiety states, infectious diseases and so on and these will hopefully be dealt with in a future volume.

The book is designed to accompany a course; mutual learning by nurses and by nurses with doctors, will add another important dimension to this project. However, the book should stand alone and I can think of few practices or few practice nurses who will not benefit from it. It is written by members of both professions and what, I think, comes through most strongly is that we are a partnership of people with a shared goal, and if we can keep up this relationship the future is bright for both disciplines in family medicine. Most of all, patient care will be that much better. I wish this book well and commend its ideals.

Michael Drury
October 1989

List of Authors

Elizabeth Armstrong was formerly the facilitator for the Heart and Stroke Prevention Project for Basingstoke and North Hants Health Authority. She now lives in Southern Italy.

Greta Barnes has been involved in promoting the development of the practice nurse's role in caring for people with asthma in recent years. She is well known for her work as Course Director of the Asthma Society Training Centre in Stratford upon Avon. She also works as a nurse in a local practice.

Elaine Fullard has been a health visitor and Health Education Officer and pioneered the role of the primary care nurse facilitator in the Oxford Prevention of Heart Attack and Stroke Project. She now has a national brief to encourage and support the appointment of other facilitators.

Peter Havelock is a general practitioner and course organizer in Bourne End, Bucks. He has developed ways of assessing and teaching communication skills in general practice and has published widely on this theme. Over the past three years he has become closely involved with facilitating the Wycombe Primary Care Prevention Project.

Richard Hobbs is a general practitioner in inner city Birmingham and a senior lecturer in the Department of General Practice at Birmingham University. He is involved in both undergraduate and postgraduate medical education and has published regularly in journals. He was one of the team who piloted and evaluated early Practice Nurse Programmes.

Phyllis Moore is a nurse practitioner who qualified at the University of California. She now works in a general practice in London. Her previous experience has included an extended nursing role in an accident and emergency department.

Ellen Murray is a nurse working in a general practice with Richard Hobbs. She has been involved with the promoting of the Practice Nurse Programme in Birmingham, and is the publicity representative for the West Midlands Practice Nurse Association.

Theo Schofield is a general practitioner in Oxfordshire and HEA lecturer in primary care at Oxford University. He has had a long interest in health teaching in general practice, and in developing communication skills with general practitioners. He works in a large general practice, and has a commitment to furthering teamwork in that setting, and nationally as chairman of Anticipatory Care Teams (ACT).

Barbara Stilwell works as a primary health care researcher for West Lambeth Health Authority. She has been involved in recent years with researching and developing the role of nurses in general practice, and, was one of the team who designed and piloted the first Practice Nurse Programme at the Department of General Practice, Birmingham.

Lilian Vincent is a nurse in general practice with Theo Schofield. She has worked on developing the shared care of people with hypertension in that practice, and is a founder member of the West Midlands Practice Nurse Association.

Preface

THIS book was initially conceived as an independent textbook for nurses working in general practice. However, a course for practice nurses which was piloted at the Department of General Practice, Birmingham University has influenced both the design and content of the book and it has now emerged as the course book for a new education package for practice nurses in England and Wales, launched in late 1989 as the practice nurse programme (PNP). Nevertheless, the book should stand alone as a reference text for practising nurses in the community, a group of specialists for whom there is at present only a limited choice of material.

The subjects have been chosen because research has shown that most practice nurses are interested in them (Stilwell and Drury 1988). Inevitably, some compromise has decided the final choice of topics and there are important omissions. Subjects not covered in this book which are relevant to practice nursing have been identified and should form the basis for a second volume. We hope this will be published alongside a complimentary course programme (PNP 2). The topics included in this book cover the principal areas of nurse input into primary care: health promotion and disease prevention; management of chronic disease; and first aid. It is also hoped that the book will provoke questions about teamwork, personal skills and the fundamental requirements for good communication. The authors who were invited to produce material, are either nationally recognized as innovators in the field or doctor and nurse teams operating together in practices. Most of the contributions have been written either by a nurse alone or by a doctor and nurse jointly. This format is important because it parallels some of the uncertainty which nursing, as a profession, has about practice nursing (Greenfield et al. 1988): what is the nursing role in the context of general practice?

BY using different contributors on the same subject, we hope that the contribution of both professions to primary care can be examined. Practising nurses may disagree with the authors and feel that their role is more or less involved than that described. Such dissent may be salutary, making you reflect on your own role and your contribution to care. If you are reading the book as part of the course, then such issues can be raised as part of the group work in which you will be involved. There is undoubtedly an overlap between family medicine and nursing practice, as there is between many other branches of the two professions. Nurses sometimes find themselves doing jobs which doctors once did, and vice versa.

At present, nurses in the community are employees either of a general practitioner or of a district health authority. Some district nurses will, in addition, have a formal attachment to a practice. This relationship will inevitably be open to the interpretation that the nurse's role is subordinate to the doctor's. In practice this may indeed be the case. This is not inevitable, however, and it is certainly not desirable. If comprehensive primary care is to flourish, then we should pay closer attention to teamwork: roles must be seen as complementary and overlaps must be first recognized and then apportioned. No two practices are the same and negotiation on professional roles is essential. In the end this is likely to strengthen the team, not undermine it.

Nurses and doctors may resent their overlap. Most of us will recognize the feeling of having one's professional territory invaded. But we are not in competition and neither has a monopoly on primary care. Constructive teamwork is possible; the more so because the unit that delivers primary care—the practice—is small enough to offer a chance of agreeing roles.

There is little doubt that the nature of primary health care is changing. More people are living longer, many with disabilities or chronic diseases. There are more risk factors which can be identified and hopefully modified through education to improve life or prevent illness. There is an increasing awareness of how much can be done through education. There is a concern not merely to respond to illness but to prevent disease and to promote health—to improve the quality of life.

With this increasing and changing workload there are tasks that doctors and nurses are both good at, and some that one profession does better than another. There is more than enough work for both, and both are needed. We hope that this book will show some of the ways forward by identifying contributions from each profession. At the very least, it should prompt you to consider the question.

Perhaps we should also say a word about what we consider nursing has to contribute to care. Nursing is not an easy profession to analyse, and sometimes its contribution to care is hard to pin down. Nursing takes account of the whole person. It pays attention to all aspects of a person— physical, mental, social and emotional—and considers the ways in which an illness affects each of these areas of life. Nursing aims to help people attain or regain the lifestyles to which they aspire. Nursing assessments should therefore take account of all these aspects of living, and nursing care plans must reflect the opinion and participation of the patient.

This book should help to answer many queries and provide the stimulus to establish new skills. It should also raise questions about how we structure care. We hope you will feel it worthwhile to go on and consider your role in more depth, and that this book will help you to begin.

Richard Hobbs
Barbara Stilwell
October 1989

References

Stilwell, B. & Drury, V. W. M. (1988) Description and evaluation of a course for practice nurses. *Journal of the Royal College of General Practitioners*, **38**, 203 – 206.

Greenfield, S. M., Stilwell, B. & Drury, V. W. M. (1988) Practice nurses: social and occupational characteristics. *Journal of the Royal College of General Practitioners*, **37**, 341 – 345.

1 The Developing Role of the Practice Nurse in Great Britain

THIS section deals with the professional development of practice nurses. There are many references listed so that interested nurses can read the research studies first hand.

Since 1966, general practitioners have been entitled to a 70% reimbursement of the salary paid to a nurse employed by them to work in the surgery. Such nurses are known as practice nurses. At the same time, other ancillary staff salaries became 70% reimbursable, and doctors were encouraged not only to employ extra staff, but also to work together in health centres employing one team between several doctors.

Other incentives were given at that time to encourage partnership arrangements and upgrading of premises. The subsidy was made following a time of great unrest amongst general practitioners, who felt that they were seriously overworked, with too many patients on their lists, and certainly felt they were underpaid. It was envisaged that a nurse working alongside a doctor might relieved him of mundane tasks, as well as broadening the scope of services available in general practice (Anderson 1973).

At the same time, delegation from doctor to nurse was encouraged by revised National Health Service terms of service for family doctors. These stated that:

> If reasonable steps are taken to ensure continuity of treatment the practitioner shall be under no obligation to give treatment personally and such treatment may be given by . . . a partner, assistant or deputy . . . or if it is reasonable in the circumstances to delegate to a member of his staff, being a person who is competent to carry out such treatment . . .

Most studies which have described the roles of practice nurses since the mid-sixties have been undertaken by doctors and have concerned various aspects of delegation of tasks (Bowling 1985). Some delegation has been extensive. One practice studied the effects of a nurse undertaking home visits (Weston-Smith & Mottram 1967; Weston-Smith & O'Donovan 1970), while Reedy (1972) noted that some practive nurses performed venepunctures, sutured wounds, gave simple physiotherapy and assessed patients attending surgery without an appointment.

Some writers have alluded to the nurse's role as listener or counsellor (Cartwright & Scott 1961; Reedy 1972) although no attempt has been made to assess the importance of these functions to patients.

Most recently, Greenfield, Stilwell and Drury (1987) sent postal questionnaries to 514 nurses from the West Midlands, of whom 300 (58%) responded. The nurses were asked to describe the work they did, and to indicate which of a list of problems they currently managed, or thought they could with extra training. They were also asked to rate the importance of several aspects of their work, in the order of priority which they felt appropriate to their roles. Most nurses currently performed conventional nursing tasks such as measurement of blood pressure, suture removal, giving injections and applying dressings. Many had a more extensive role since over 70% took cervical smears, 62% examined breasts and 69% undertook auroscopic examination of the ears, nose and throat. Only a few had roles extended into conventional medical areas, with 8% of nurses using a stethoscope to examine the heart and chest and 4% carrying out abdominal palpation. Overall, 82% of nurses felt that practical tasks were the most important aspect of their work, and preventive and screening procedures came second. Sixty per cent of nurses thought that advising patients about coping with illness was of only moderate importance in their work. Counselling patients also ranked of moderate importance (67%); and 69% of nurses thought their role was extended beyond that of basic training. There were enormous variations in the patterns of work of this sample of practice nurses, highlighting a lack of role definition.

Others have expressed concern at the practice nurses' role possibly deserting the caring ethic of nursing in favour of delegated medical tasks (Skeet 1978; Hockey 1984). Certainly, in the West Midlands sample of nurses, practice tasks (some of them taken over from doctors) were the most important aspect of their work. It is probably the extension of the nursing role into these traditionally medical areas which has led some authors to compare the role of the practice nurse with that of the American nurse practitioner (Devlin 1985), and in some practices nurses are now employed with the title of nurse practitioner.

Interestingly, Reddy (1980) in a study of 153 practice nurses' activities and opinions said:

> There is . . . a close analogy between the role and organisational position of the employed nurse in Britain and the physician's assistant in America . . . It remains to be seen if [the nurses'] apparent acceptance of technical activities becomes associated with the dependence on doctors which characterizes the physician's assistant role . . .

How close has the practice nurse come to the nurse practitioner or physician's assistant?

Nurse practitioners in British general practice

A recent study by Stilwell *et al.* (1987) describes what happened when a specially trained nurse practitioner was introduced into an inner city general practice. The nurse practitioner (a woman) worked with one female and two male doctors, and patients had free access to nurse practitioner care.

The nurse worked in a consulting room similar to that of the doctors. Patients were offered 20-minute appointments and were advised of the nurse practitioner's presence by a large notice in the waiting room which described the nurse as having further training in the management of common family health problems. Consultations were informal, patients being encouraged to talk about themselves and their lifestyles. Health teaching was held to be an important component of nursing practice (Stilwell 1985). This extended time given to each patient was found, in a pilot project, to be necessary for an adequate nursing assessment and to incorporate relevant health teaching (Stilwell 1982). The aim of each consultation was to deal with the presenting problem, taking into account factors other than physical symptoms, and focus on long-term health education.

Analysis of the work of the nurse practitioner over a 6-month period showed that the majority of people consulting her were women. Most people were under 40 years of age, and over half had chosen to consult her. The majority of problems presented to the nurse practitioner (60%) concerned social and emotional problems or health education.

These findings support that of Chen *et al.* (1984) who evaluated the work of an American nurse practitioner in an ambulatory care setting and found that she saw a higher proportion of women than did the doctors. Similarly, most of the problems they encountered were not related to disease or injury but to social and emotional problems or health education. No outcome measures were attempted for the work of this British nurse practitioner study, but it was possible to say that there was no evidence of serious disorders going unnoticed. It was found that the nurse practitioner managed the patient's presenting problem without referral, prescription or investigation in 45% of all cases. This suggests that consultations were appropriate for nursing care alone, and were chosen appropriately by patients.

Comparisons of practice nurse and nurse practitioner's work

Have practice nurses developed roles similar to those of an American nurse practitioner? The Birmingham nurse practitioner study was based on the

American model, and perhaps for that reason showed similar trends in outcome measures and content of work. MacGuire (1980) said that:

> Nurses here are quietly expanding their roles . . . to meet new demands without an accompanying fanfare of new titles. Let us not be misled into thinking that in adopting 'nurse practitioners' we would be introducing anything new.

Many believe this to be true, and yet without a role definition for either a practice nurse or a nurse practitioner, it is quite impossible to make such a statement. What it is possible to say is that the role of the practice nurse has been changing, and is still changing.

Rather than comparing two roles which have no definition, it is perhaps more helpful to think of the role of the nurse in general practice as running along a continuum from a nurse who accepts delegated tasks, to one who acts as an autonomous professional. Table 1.1 illustrates this continuum through several areas of practice.

Table 1.1   Comparison of extended and limited roles for a practice nurse.

Extended role	Limited role
Collect information in wide field (physical examination, including investigations) Sorting information	Collect information in narrow field Minimal sorting of information
Have complex presentations	Have simple presentations
Are able to help patient make decision about nursing interventions	Not involved in decision-making, refer to doctor
Incorporates supportive role in nursing	Minimal supportive strategies
Takes pain to promote understanding in consultations	Traditional health education methods
Plans (organizes) own work	Plans work according to others' demands/needs
Establishes a relationship with clients	Carries on the doctor's relationship with a client
Understands the importance of social skills	Social skills are hit and miss

What should nurses in general practice be doing?

This question calls for answers to two important considerations for nurses: What is the unique contribution which nurses can make to primary health care? What are nurses good at?

The problem for British practice nursing is that we have little evidence to answer these questions. Perhaps the best research studies which indicate a nurse's potential contribution to health care come from American studies on nurse practitioner care. Outcomes of nurse practitioner care in America have been extensively evaluated (Molde & Diers 1985). There is now considerable evidence that nurse practitioners provide care which is safe and sometimes more effective than that of some physicians (Sullivan 1982). It is, however, unhelpful only to compare nurse practitioners with physicians because it simply serves to highlight their overlapping roles.

In developing the practice nurse's role it is important to acknowledge that their scope of practice *will* develop with that of physicians, but the emphasis for nurses must be different. The emphasis of their role is not primarily on diagnosis and treatment, but is concerned both to help people understand and cope with illness or early signs of illness, and to be supportive to those who cannot cope. A recent unpublished study by Stilwell examined the attitudes of people consulting practice nurses and found that there were three reasons why the majority of people did so.

1 They felt that the nurse had time for them.
2 They felt they could just pop in and talk over 'trivial' problems.
3 They felt the nurse cared about them.

This supports earlier findings, when Anderson (1973) reported that nurses were expected to be kind, understanding, patient, sympathetic, cheerful and available to the patient. They were also expected to provide emotional support. (A further finding from this study was that doctors expected nurses to be technically competent, rather than to provide emotional support. This is an apparent paradox, which it would be interesting to explore—but that is another chapter.)

It seems that the potential of what nurses can do lies in the relationship established between the nurse and the client. This has its foundations in the client expectations that the nurse will understand and be sympathetic. It is within this relationship that health teaching can begin. If people trust the nurse to be supportive, they will ask 'trivial' questions and will 'admit' to unhealthy lifestyle practices.

Most practice nurses will acknowledge that a large part of their work is concerned with health education. Indeed, there is an increasing trend to employ nurses to help with a practice's preventive work.

American studies show that nurse practitioners have excellent outcomes in helping people change their lifestyles. One study showed that hypertensive people cared for by nurse practitioners had better blood pressure control than when they had been cared for by physicians (Ramsay *et al.* 1982). Another found that nurse practitioners were effective at helping people lose weight, keep appointments and comply with recommendations (Watkins & Wagner 1982). A British study showed similar results (Kenkre *et al.* 1985) when a nurse cared for hypertensive people in three general practices. What no-one understands is why nurses have such good outcomes in the field of care of chronic disorders or lifestyle counselling. It may be related to the quality of the relationship between nurse and client. Research is needed to establish this link.

In summary then, it seems that nurses are good at counselling people toward healthier lifestyles and have potential access to many people coming into the primary health care system. If this is what nurses are (or can be) good at, then this is what nurses should be doing.

The importance of research

There has been much speculation in this chapter about what practice nurses are doing, what they are good at doing and whether they should be doing it. These are all research questions.

It has been said that nursing is not a profession because it does not have a research base underpinning its practice. That has certainly been true in the past, but is changing in many areas of nursing. Practice nursing remains under-researched. There is no reason why practice nurses should not undertake small research projects based on their work. Many practices are near a university where research expertise is available to guide nurses through research processes. The following could be considered.

1   What are the outcomes of nursing care in general practice?
2   What processes do nurses use?
3   How do practice nurses set standards?
4   How does change come about in nursing practice?

These are fundamental questions for practice nurses, and urgently need answers if a role is to be developed which maximizes the potential of nursing to improve the quality of primary health care.

The importance of education

The Cumberledge Report (Department of Health & Social Security 1986) did practice nurses a big favour. It pointed out that practice nurses were inadequately educationally prepared for their jobs. In fact, studies of practice nurses' social and occupational characteristics have shown that they are likely to have returned to nursing after a break of several years for family commitments. This means that in the past, practice nurses have been employed following a long break in career, and without educational updating.

Furthermore, once employed in practice many practice nurses have been 'trained' by their doctor colleague to do tasks. The Cumberledge Report considered that doctors should not educate nurses. The results of these criticisms, whether right or wrong, has been to galvanize practice nurses into action, and courses for practice nurses are proliferating. They do not always meet practice nurse educational needs, partly because there are so few practice nurses on academic staffs.

Clearly, there will be a need for educators to come from the professional branch of practice nursing, as well as practical work teachers based in practice. In the end, they can be no substitute for formal education. It is to be hoped that a qualification will be developed which will demonstrate excellence in practice nursing.

The past and the future

We discuss the future in Chapter 9, so will not write about it now—except to say that there *is* a future for nursing in family practice. Nurses have much to congratulate themselves on and yet they seldom do so, they are often content to sit back and let their skills go unacknowledged. Nursing in general, and practice nursing in particular, contributes uniquely to patient care. Because it does so, it should be rewarded for its importance, both in terms of respect and money.

The past provides an interesting story. The morals to be drawn centre around professional self-respect, confidence and responsibilities. The earliest record of a nurse employed by a general practitioner is in Easington, Northumberland in 1913 called Mary Hannah Robson (N. Brown 1987, personal communication).

> Her duties were varied. She would assist Dr Grant in his surgery, helping with dressings and even doing dispensing from stock bottles . . . She lived in the practice house with the Grant family and her bedroom window overlooked the front door so that when the night bell rang, she could take any messages. Evidently she used to vet these night calls and if she could deal with them she went to see them herself. Other calls were passed on to the doctor. She often visited the Ambulance Room at the local pit to see injured miners. It was no trouble to poultice a case of pleurisy or pneumonia and she used to tell about her treatment of a miner's greyhound which required 26 stitches in a laceration . . .

Brown goes on to say that Miss Robson acted as a doctor surrogate during the 1914 – 18 war, visiting patients in nearby villages. Clearly this practice nurse took on a considerably extended role though she apparently remained subordinate in status. In 1947 she earned £221-4-11d compared with the doctor's £2406-4-11d.

References

Anderson, E. (1973) *The Role of the Nurse.* Royal College of Nurses, London.

Bowling, A. (1985) Delegation and substitution. In *Health Care UK,* (eds A. Hamson & J. Gretton). Chartered Institute of Public Finance and Accountancy, London.

Cartwright, A. & Scott, R. (1961) The work of a nurse employed in general practice. *British Medical Journal,* 1, 803 – 813.

Cater, M. L. & Hawthorn, P. J. (1987) *Survey of practice nurses in the UK—their extended roles.* Paper given at conference on Nurse Practitioners and Practice Nurses, St Bartholomew's Hospitals, London.

Chen, S. C., Barkanskas, V. H. & Chen, E. (1984) Health problems encountered by nurse practitioners and physicians in general medicine clinics. *Research in Nursing and Health,* 7, 79 – 86.

Department of Health & Social Security (1986) *Neighbourhood Nursing: A Focus for Care.* Report of the Community Nursing Review, HMSO, London.

Greenfield, S., Stilwell, B. & Drury, V. W. M. (1987) Practice nurses: social and occupational characteristics. *Journal of the Royal College of General Practitioners,* 37, 341 – 345.

Hockey, L. (1984) Is the practice nurse a good idea? *Journal of the Royal College of General Practitioners,* 34, 102 – 103.

Kenkre, J., Drury, V. W. M. & Lancashire, R. J. (1985) Nurse management of hypertension clinics in general practice, assisted by a computer. *Family Practice,* 2(1), 17 – 22.

MacGuire, J. M. (1980) *The Expanded Role of the Nurse.* Kings College Fund, London.

Molde, S. & Diers, D. (1985) Nurse practitioner research: selected literature review and research agenda. *Nursing Research,* 34, 362 – 367.

Ramsay, J., Mckenzie, J. & Fish, D. (1982) Physicians and nurse practitioners: do they provide equal health care? *American Journal of Public Health,* 72, 55 – 57.

Reedy, B. L. E. C. (1972) Organisation and management: the general practice nurse. *Update,* 5, 75 – 78.

Reedy, B. L. E. C. (1980) A comparison of the activities and opinions of attached and employed nurses in general practice. *Journal of The Royal College of General Practitioners,* 30, 483 – 489.

Skeet, M. (1978) Health auxiliaries: decision makers and implementer. In *Health Auxilliaries and the Health Team,* (eds M. Skeet & R. Elliot). Croom Helm, London.

Stilwell, B. (1982) The nurse practitioner at work. 1 Primary care. *Nursing Times,* 78, 1799 – 1803.

Stilwell, B. (1985) Prevention and health: the concern of nursing. *Journal of The Royal College of General Practitioners*, **105**, 60 – 62.

Stilwell, B. Greenfield, S., Drury, V. W. M. & Hull, F. M. (1987) A nurse practitioner in general practice: working styles and pattern of consultations. *Journal of The Royal College of General Practitioners*, **37**, 154 – 157.

Sullivan, J. (1982) Research on nurse practitioners: process behind the outcome? *American Journal of Public Health*, **72**, 8 – 9.

Watkins, L. & Wagner, E. (1982) Nurse practitioner and physician adherence to standing orders criteria for consultations as referral. *American Journal of Public Health*, **72**, 22 – 29.

Weston-Smith, J. & Mottram, E. M. (1967) Extended use of nursing service in general practice. *British Medical Journal*, **4**, 672 – 672.

Weston-Smith, J. & O'Donovan, J. B. (1970) The practice nurse—a new look. *British Medical Journal*, **4**, 673 – 677.

Further reading

Bowling, A. & Stilwell, B. (1988) *The Nurse in Family Practice*. Sintari Press, London.

2 General Practice and the Primary Care Team

GENERAL practice is structured, funded and organized in a way that is quite separate from the rest of the health service. This historical legacy has contributed to many of the general practice's successes but has also led to some notable deficiencies. Futhermore, simply because it is different, its methods and priorities are frequently misunderstood by other sections of the medical and nursing establishment. This chapter will discuss briefly how the general practice functions within the National Health Service (NHS). Such information will be particularly useful to nurses who are new to practice nursing or are working as attached employees of the district health authority (DHA). The roles of other members of a primary care team are also discussed.

Delivery of comprehensive preventive and reactive primary health care requires an organized team approach. When it operates smoothly, there is no better example of multidisciplinary teamwork than that seen in general practice.

Structure of the National Health Service

The National Health Service Act of 1946 charged the Minister of Health with the responsibility to establish a service providing all patients, free of charge, with all the necessities for the prevention, diagnosis and treatment of illness. In practical terms the organization that resulted was an amalgamation of existing disparate services into three main areas: provision for the sick in institutions, provision for the sick in the community, and prevention of sickness. The three main service branches were correspondingly the hospital services, general practitioner (GP) services and the local health authority services.

The main service provision from the hospital side of the NHS is at district health authority (DHA) level. The DHA is also the main point of contact between general practitioners and the hospital sector. As well as providing secondary and occasionally tertiary care services in the local hospital, the DHA is responsible for:

- maternity and child health service;
- health visiting;
- community nursing (district nurse and midwife);

- immunizations;
- community health clinics (family planning, chiropody);
- health centres;
- health education;
- school health;
- ambulance service.

The NHS Act saw a fundamental change in the structure of general practice. Previously this had been a disorganized service. Doctors principally earned either private fees or salaries from large working organizations such as coal mining committees. Inevitably there were great variations between GP incomes and between the distribution of their practices throughout the United Kingdom. Most doctors were single-handed, with a few in groups of two or rarely three.

With the establishment of the NHS, general practitioners virtually entirely replaced their private incomes with a standard capital fee attracted with each patient registered with the doctor. The GP was not actually employed by the NHS, but subcontracted his time (normally all of it) to the service. The organizing body was the Executive Council which was equivalent in geographical responsibility to the DHA. In 1974, this became the Family Practitioner Committee (FPC). This change not only provided every patient with the possibility of a GP, but it also, with the advice of the Medical Practices Committee (MPC), distributed GPs equitably around the country depending on the existing density of family doctors.

The FPC is solely responsible for:

- administering the contracts of doctors, dentists, chemists and opticians;
- arranging for duly claimed payments;
- conducting disciplinary procedures if the terms and conditions of service are breached.

The composition of the FPC includes 30 members, 15 lay and 15 professional, of whom eight are general practitioners elected by the Local Medical Committee (LMC), three dentists, two are pharmacists and two are opticians. This representation will entirely change should the White Paper, *Working for Patients*, be implemented. The principal change will be a reduction of the medical input to the FPC to one doctor (who need not be a GP) on a smaller committee of 12 members. At present the FPC seeks advice on all matters relating to general practice from the LMC. This is a body of regularly elected GPs who represent their colleagues from an area co-terminous with the FPC. This route for advice will also end with the White Paper.

Over the years the structure of general practice has altered considerably. Most doctors now practice in groups (Figure 2.1). Premises have dramatically improved in the past 10 – 15 years. Both of these changes were

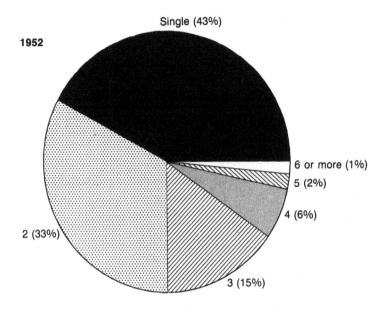

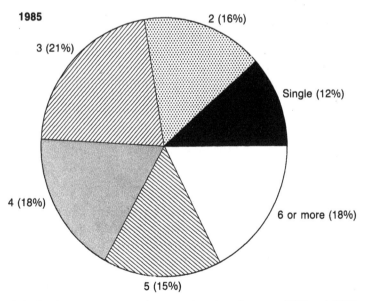

Fig. 2.1 Single and group practice—a comparison between 1952 and 1985.

promoted by special incentives to help practices join up and by cost/rent/improvement grants for building renovation. Sixty per cent of doctors own their surgery premises, 25% practise from a health centre (60% in Northern Ireland), and only 15% rent accommodation.

However, perhaps the greatest impact on the efficiency of general practice has been made by the introduction of two factors—the direct reimbursement of staff (discussed on p. 15) and vocational training. Since 1981, it has been compulsory for doctors to complete additional specialist training before entry into general practice. Vocational training regulations stipulate that following the 12-month, pre-registration house jobs, aspiring GPs should spend a minimum of 2 years in further hospital training from a selection of relevant specialities including medicine, paediatrics, psychiatry, geriatrics, accident and emergency (A & E), obstetrics, and gynaecology. A further 12 months is spent as a trainee in a special training practice.

At a time when general practice is the most popular first choice for a medical career, the experience of vocational training has helped to ensure that future GPs are more adequately prepared for their role.

Financing of general practice and the NHS

Arrangements for funding general practice are complicated and because practices are required to operate with fiscal efficiency, GPs have earned perhaps an undeserved reputation for being businessmen. Since they are not directly employed by the NHS, family doctors do not earn salaries. They are required to make direct claims to the FPC for services provided or necessary expenses. These FPC payments collectively make up the gross income to the practice. Most will also have some private income from insurance medicals, report and the like, but this will be a very small component (under 5%) for the majority.

Income from the FPC is broadly divided into four areas.

1 *Basic practice allowance*

Each full time principal who satisfies minimum criteria laid out in the terms and conditions of service will receive this payment. It is intended to cover on call. This fixed figure is totally representative of actual costs since it is arrived at by analysing the expenses claimed against tax in a proportion of Inland Revenue returns from practices.

2 *Capitation fees and registration*

Capitation fees are standard rates attracted by the presence of each patient on the doctor's list. It is expected that a minumum level of services will be offered to the patient. For example, the fee of £8.95 per year which is presently paid for a patient under 65 (1989 prices) is to cover every basic consultation the patient receives between the hours of 7 a.m. and 11 p.m. over a 12-month period, whether at the surgery or at home. There is a slightly increased fee for patients over 65, and again over 75. There are certain additional payments made for temporary, emergency or night visits (11 p.m. – 7 a.m.).

3   Direct expense reimbursement

The rent and rates on practice premises which have been agreed by the FPC are reimbursed in full. Ancillary staff salaries are covered up to a level of 70% (and 100% of their National Insurance contributions are paid) for a maximum of two full time staff per GP principal. Only certain positions are allowable under this scheme and these include receptionists, practice managers and nurses. Counsellors and physiotherapists are not recognized by most FPCs.

4   Items of service payments

Certain activities performed in practice attract separate payments. Since the NHS had originally intended that general practice simply provided for sick people in the community, when more preventive activities were expected of them a new payment system was evolved. Items of service fees are therefore payable for antenatal care, advice on contraceptive services, certain cervical smears (women over 35 years, every 5 years) and some immunizations and vaccinations (all childhood, some adult immunizations and recommended travel vaccinations).

Approximately one-third of income comes from source 1, one-third from 2, and the final third from 3 and 4. All these claimed payments make up the practice income from which all practice expenses are financed, including all the staff salaries, heating and lighting, equipment, rent or maintenance. Any money left over (the practice profit) is divided amongst the GP partners according to their agreed shares. The review body, which advises the government on the salaries of doctors, sets a figure each year which it intends that GPs should earn after practice expenses have been deducted.

Only receiving income for what is claimed and personally managing income and expenditure within the team that actually provides the service is an unusual arrangement. It does tend to promote financial prudence. This is one of the factors which contributes to the low overall cost of general practice to the NHS annual bill. Despite providing for 93% of all medical consultations in the UK, and employment for half the doctors, general practice consumes only 6% of the NHS budget. This 6% includes every payment made by the FPC for fees and staff/premises reimbursements. If the drugs bill is added to this total, expenditure rises to around 13%. This low level is despite the fact that some 95% of all drugs are now prescribed by GPs as hospitals have transferred their drug costs onto the community sector.

This relatively small percentage expenditure on primary care has to be further set against the overall low level of funding of the whole health service. Britain continues to spend substantially less on the health of its population than other developed countries. Indeed, using percentage expenditure of the gross national product (GNP), or the country's wealth, we are the most miserly providers in the developed world (see Figures 2.2 and 2.3), spending a lower proportion on health than even an impoverished country like Turkey.

Although expenditure on private medicine has increased, particularly in recent years (now 10% of what is spent on the NHS), this continues to provide only a tiny fraction of the actual activities that occur in the health service (less than 1%).

Ancillary staff

The nucleus of the primary care team is the ancillary practice staff, whose roles are briefly discussed here.

Practice manager

This is the senior administrative staff member with special responsibilites for:

- planning services;
- managing the most efficient use of accommodation and equipment;
- advising on systems for the smooth running of surgeries and emergencies;
- financial administration/preparation of practice accounts;
- liaison with accountant;
- training of reception staff;
- responsibility for statutory returns;
- co-ordinating data collection and statistics;
- liaising with other health service staff;
- dealing with visitors.

There is no traditional career route for practice managers. Many will have worked up from secretarial positions within practices, gaining the necessary skills 'on the job'. However, the pressure for more uniform

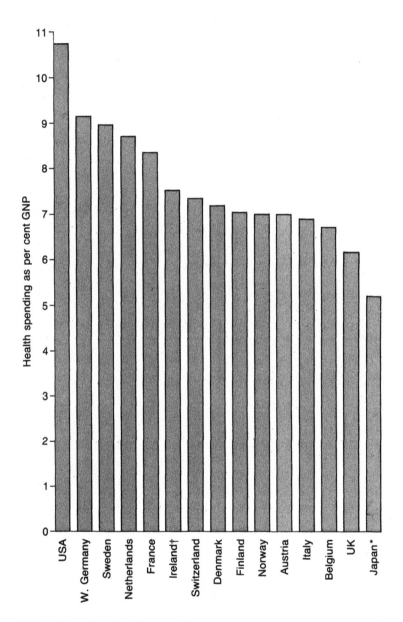

* Excluding private health expenditure.

† Excluding capital expenditure.

Fig. 2.2   Health care spending expressed as per cent GNP in selected
OECD countries, 1984.

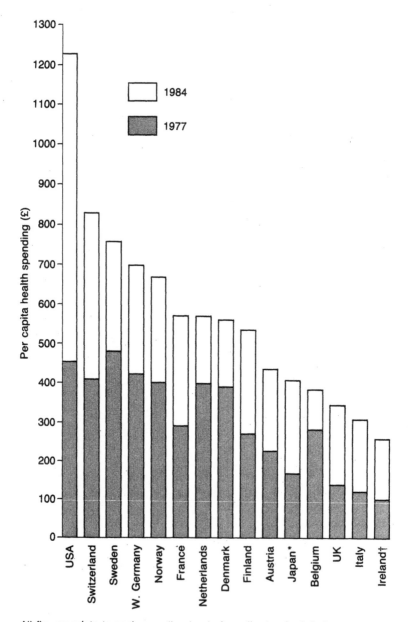

All figures relate to cash spending i.e. before allowing for inflation.

* Excluding private health expenditure.

† Excluding capital expenditure.

Fig. 2.3   Health spending per head of population in selected OECD countries, 1977 and 1984.

training has led to a variety of courses around the country, including those run by AMSPAR and PMD courses organized by Radcliffe Medical Press. A group practice of four doctors might well have a gross turnover of over £250 000, a clear indication of the responsibilities of a practice manager.

Receptionists/medical secretaries

The image of the receptionist will often provide a measure of the practice. Receptionists' principal functions include all or some of the following:

- organizing the flow of patients in surgery;
- acting as telephonists;
- answering patient queries;
- filtering requests to the doctors;
- maintaining patient record files;
- preparing claims for the FPC;
- arranging for repeat prescriptions;
- recording practice statistics on workload.

Their role is frequently a difficult one since they are the most accessible member of the practice. There is a fine balance between being obstructive to waiting patients and preventing too many interruptions for patients during consultation. It is ultimately the doctor's responsibility to ensure that receptionists are adequately trained for this difficult role and the image projected by reception staff is usually one to which the GPs subscribe. The most successful reception staff training is the Practice Receptionist Programme (PRP) organized by the Radcliffe Medical Press.

Inevitably many of the roles of receptionists will also be performed by secretaries. Additional priorities are:

- letters and reports;
- arranging hospital referrals;
- maintaining manual card index systems;
- possibly organizing calls and recalls;
- computer data entry.

Practice nurses

The role of the practice nurse has expanded rapidly in its brief history. Perhaps inevitably, in some practices their duties are limited to such matters as dressings, ear syringing, cervical cytology, immunizations and the taking of blood specimens. However, there is great potential for role enhancement and, this is the stimulus for this book.

Attached staff

Community nurses

At present around 80% of all district health authority community nurses, health visitors and midwives are practice attached. However, geographical or patch attachment is increasing following the recommendations of the Cumberledge Report on the future of community nursing. There are many convincing arguments on both sides, but for the primary health care team to operate with most effect, regard has to be given to some kind of named person/named practice attachment.

Midwife clinics operating in tandem with antenatal clinics will usually achieve high patient uptake even in inner city areas. Parentcraft and relaxation classes are ideally organized in these deprived practices where lack of access to cheap travel is likely to deter hospital visits.

Health visitor involvement in antenatal and paediatric development clinics has obvious benefits and is also extremely cost effective with good access to a captive audience. It is sobering to reflect that health visitors spend over a third of their working time in travelling between patients. Close consultation between the health visitor and practice is particularly beneficial in difficult cases like abuse or neglect, where information from several sources may enable action to be taken more quickly in sudden crises.

Assuming that the practice nurse is prepared to take on some of the district nurse duties with patients who can get to the surgery, more time is released for the district nurse to concentrate on home visiting.

A welcome development in the past 10 years has been the establishment of community psychiatric nurses (CPNs). Many of these have formal practice attachments and arrange counselling clinics in the surgery, as well as monitoring the psychiatrically ill in the community and arranging depot injection clinics. Their closer links with practices have frequently led to admissions being easier to arrange for the severely ill, particularly if they are compulsory detentions under a section of the Mental Health Act.

Other health professionals

Social workers should ideally form part of every primary care team. Unfortunately, major contractions in social services expenditure have severely reduced their numbers. Their particular skills lie in advice on benefits and disability services, housing, sheltered accommodation, and follow-up of children on at-risk registers. Some will provide counselling support in clinics.

Responsibilities for the mentally ill are now vested in designated psychiatric social workers who receive special intensive training. They liaise closely with CPNs and hospital psychiatric services.

The ideal practice team would also have a close liaison with dietitians, physiotherapists, occupational therapists, orthoptists, counsellors, speech therapists, marriage guidance, continence services and special aids. Unfortunately, many of these services are readily available only to practices in health authority premises, where the community staff are also based. However, other practices should not be discouraged from attempting to forge links.

Teamwork

It would be comforting to hope that a collection of health workers in general practice with multidisciplinary roles would automatically operate as a primary health care team. Unfortunately, this cannot be relied on since the concept of a team involves a common approach to agreed goals, and this requires a personal and active commitment from each member. Ultimately the goals for all health workers are the prevention of illness, improvement of ill health and palliation of symptoms. It is the method of achieving these which challenges agreement within teams. The most critical ingredient for successful teams is therefore adequate communication between members. This is more likely to take place if team meetings feature regularly in the practice timetable.

Team meetings

The team meeting has an important socializing role in helping members relate more comfortably to each other. The importance of this should not be underestimated since a team approach to health care requires a liberal quantity of trust. As long as the meetings operate with certain basic rules, the development of trust should take place. These rules should include:

- respect for each other's special skills;
- support for team approach;
- personal involvement in the negotiation of team objectives;
- acceptance of the consensus view.

A good way of facilitating the group process in early team meetings is to choose to work on a clinical task which has the personal interest of most members. This might be, for example, to improve immunization or cervical smear rates or to develop a standard protocol for managing diabetes or hypertension. This is not to suggest that the task itself is necessarily easy, but choosing a topic that is solidly clinical and important would be more likely to attract involvement of the group, both in negotiation and implementation. A successful first task should boost confidence in the relevance of teamwork. Areas to cover in task-orientated meetings should include:

- agreeing common objectives;
- negotiating roles;
- allocating responsibilities;
- measuring some element of outcome;
- feedback of progress at future meetings;
- formulating management plan (protocol).

Once a successful format for the team meetings has been established, a regular timetable must be followed. It may be necessary to offer certain groups additional discussions. This is particularly true for practice employed staff who may want the opportunity to discuss grievances or resolve an organizational problem.

For teamwork to succeed an investment in team support is crucial. For those whose primary function lies outside the practice, involvement in a discrete practice group may be politically sensitive. Discussion with the District Unit General Manager can assist co-operation. Managers might even be invited to become involved with relevant meetings should the district policy be out of step with agreed practice objectives. The final composition and regularity of team meetings is a matter for individual practices to debate.

It is taken for granted that members of a practice will be talking with each other during the normal course of their duties. Formal meetings will in no way replace this important source of information sharing. However, to ensure that the processes discussed so far take place, certain additional details should be incorporated. Meetings time should occur at a regular time, on a regular day. If attempts are made to organize meetings when everyone can attend they will not take place. At least some meetings should be open to *all* members of the team. Some disciplines might require additional meetings particularly if there is to be an educational input. An agenda should always be prepared and all points on the agenda should be covered, if necessary by an additional meeting. Finally, the team should be prepared to invite temporary members if a new initiative is taking place which crosses practice boundaries.

The practice meeting can therefore perform several functions, some simultaneously, others only occasionally. These will include:

- improving team relationships;
- facilitating structured primary care;
- prevention, early diagnosis, call/recall systems;
- chronic disease and drug review;
- planning future health developments;

- discussing practice evolution;
- resolving grievances;
- continuing medical/nursing/administrative education;
- multidisciplinary medical audit;
- multidisciplinary peer support.

The designated team meeting should provide an efficient, motivating force for constructive change in the practice's delivery of health care. Without dedicated time for discussion, negotiation and decision, progress forward is likely to be slow, patchy or ineffectual.

Audit

The purpose of the teamwork discussed so far has been to produce the strategy for improved delivery of health care. A necessary follow-on from this is some measure of outcome: Has the strategy produced the desired result? Audit is the method by which we examine what we do. Unfortunately it is a rather inexact term with connotations of external scrutiny and crude targets. It strictly derives from the Latin word for 'hearing', in an active sense. This is an activity that most of us would feel is a very important skill for health workers. Just as we should consult in a way which enables us to 'hear' for the hidden patient agenda, so we should audit what we practice, since the reality may not accord with what we think takes place.

In a sense, the overriding conclusion from this view of audit is that we should all incorporate it automatically into the way we practice. We should be concerned as to whether our intentions translate into deeds. If audit is an activity that becomes automatic, then its implementation should become that much easier. Once again, the team meeting is a good starting point to build in some measurement of outcome into agreed policies. A simple example would be to calculate the practice completed immunization rates for 12-month-olds (triple), 20-month-olds (MMR—measles, mumps and rubella) and 5-year-olds (pre-school booster). This could act as a stimulus to develop strategies for improvement. Any change could be measured by regular audit of the rates. Strategies could then be reviewed and altered if no change had occurred.

A more complicated example of audit might be the measurement of clinical protocols that were in operation. A hypertensive audit would need various measurements: Had the at-risk group been screened? Were abnormal readings followed up? Were the drugs prescribed ones agreed to? Was blood pressure control adequate? Were additional risks, like smoking, followed up? This data could be collected from a random sample of patient records and the use of a hypertension disease register.

Audit can therefore provide the following benefits to the team:

- stimulus to improve practice;
- feedback on the success of practice strategies;
- test of practice disease protocols;
- provides practice statistics;
- a measure of the effectiveness of liaison between team members.

Anticipatory care

One of the principal responsibilities for the primary care team is the structured care of chronic disease. This is underlined by the inclusion of three chapters on diabetes, hypertension and asthma management in this book. However, the area of potentially greatest expansion in practice development is disease prevention and health promotion. Anticipatory care is the term that describes these two activities, to contrast with reactive care which covers the medical response to illness.

Prevention

Primary prevention of a disease aims to avoid the development of risk factors in individuals. This involves health education, for example about smoking or sensible diets; and prophylaxis, for example immunization or vaccination.

Secondary prevention aims to recognize risk factors or to detect disease at an early stage, and therefore justifies most screening programmes. By identifying disease early, remedial action can be taken which may alter prognosis, for example of certain cancers and hyperlipidaemia.

Tertiary prevention is aimed at the limitation of complications once the disease is established. This care should not be neglected by primary care teams. Indeed, only through concerted teamwork is tertiary prevention likely to operate effectively. By regular and scrupulous review, problems like retinopathy, renal failure in diabetes, or strokes and heart attacks in hypertension, might be avoided.

Screening

The practice nurse is likely to be heavily involved in primary and secondary prevention. The latter requires systems development in order to be comprehensive. The methods that are available include formal screening of patients and opportunistic case finding.

Formal screening uses call and recall of the at-risk group. This group can be identified from an age/sex register, whether manual or computer derived. Patients can be sent for and then followed-up regularly. Diseases worth screening for include cervical cytology, hypertension, and possibly glaucoma and other cancers (breast, testicular, bowel). Unfortunately, patients will demonstrate variable uptake of routinely offered screening and this is particularly true of poorer populations who paradoxically are generally at highest risk.

An alternative to formal screening is opportunistic screening or case finding. Here, the attendance of the patient with another problem prompts the offer of preventive screening as an extra. This is discussed further on p. 51. Since 65% of patients will consult their practice each year, the average being three attendances for men and four for women, screening opportunistically is both cost effective and safe. Evidence is also available to show that the GP and practice nurse are the most proficient of all health workers in producing changes in lifestyle. Diseases or risk factors particularly appropriate for opportunistic screening are hypertension, smoking, hyperlipidaemia and any non-responder to formal screening.

The adoption of anticipatory care encourages an approach to health care that is more aware and more alert to potential risk factors and early disease recognition. It aims to:

1 improve the quality of life;
2 identify potential risk factors;
3 reduce the disability of premature disease;
4 reduce the disability of established diseases;
5 prevent disease extension;
6 prolong life.

Further reading

Bowling, A. (1981) *Delegation in General Practice*. Tavistock Publications, London.
British Medical Association (1983) *Organising a Practice*. BMA, London.
Jeffreys, M. & Sachs, H. (1983) *Rethinking General Practice*. Tavistock Publications, London.
Pritchard, P. (1978) *Manual of Primary Health Care*. Oxford University Press, Oxford.
Pritchard, P., Law, K. & Whalen, M. (1984) *Management in General Practice*. Oxford University Press, Oxford.
Stott, N. C. H. (1983) *Primary Health Care: Bridging the Gap Between Theory and Practice*. Springer Verlag, Berlin.
Stott, N. C. H. & Pill, R. M. (198) *Health Checks in General Practice: Why Some People Attend and Others Do Not*. University of Wales, Cardiff.
Westcott, R. H. & Jones R. V. H. (1988) *Information Handling in General Practice: Challenges for the Future*. Croom Helm, London.

3 Communication Skills

Why bother to read this chapter?

'All experienced nurses are good communicators, so why bother to teach us what we know.'

THE above quotation came from a practice nurse in an evaluation of a communication skills course. It is certainly true that many nurses can communicate well, but does that mean they realize the value of what they do, or that they understand the potential effect of those skills? Learning how to communicate effectively is as important as learning good clinical practice, because if our patients understand what we say to them, they are more likely to follow our advice; if we relate well to our patients they are more likely to return for follow-up.

There are, at present, more than 7000 practice nurses in England. If each nurse sees only 10 patients a day, that means there are one-third of a million nurse consultations taking place in general practice every week of the year. Each consultation has the potential to be used as a means of education on health matters. With the drive towards 'Health for All' by the year 2000, it is vital to use this potential. This explains the need to foster effective communication skills. It is impossible in one chapter to teach all there is to know on the subject, but we will discuss the most important points, as well as offer a guide to further reading.

Another important element of this chapter will be the section on feeling good about yourself and managing your work environment. It is impossible to relate to others in a mature and confident way unless you first look after your own mental and emotional health. This chapter will help you to cope with difficult or demanding situations by facing up to, understanding, and describing your own feelings.

Patients, nurses and communication

When a person chooses to consult a nurse, it is often because:

- it is easier to gain access to the nurse than the doctor;
- people expect nurses to have time for them;
- nurses are expected to be kind, sympathetic and understanding.

Research has found that practice nurses are usually good communicators, but on a rather *ad hoc* basis. Practice nurses have often had no formal education or training in communication skills. They are often only responsive to evident patient needs, such as a person crying or asking for specific information. There is nothing wrong with this way of working, but its weakness is that the nurse is not necessarily aware of what she is doing, or more importantly, what she could be doing by employing certain communication skills. Perhaps the most obvious example of this unfulfilled potential is in promoting health. Teaching adults is not easy. They have acquired beliefs and prejudices which need to be uncovered before they can be changed. There are techniques which can be used to make these processes more effective, and therefore to facilitate necessary lifestyle changes.

Research into nurses' effectiveness as communicators shows that, while informal contact with patients and their relatives is made in a warm and caring way, nurses have poor formal communication skills (Kagan *et al.* 1986). Kagan *et al.* give four reasons why this may be so, stating that nurses need to:

1 develop insights into their own interpersonal skills in order to use them effectively;
2 learn how to apply interpersonal skills to their own field of work;
3 understand the use and effectiveness of particular ways of communication;
4 know the constraints to effective communication skills in clinical settings.

It is important, however, that practice nurses should not lose the warm informality which makes them accessible to their patients. Learning more about communication skills will not destroy the interpersonal skills which you already have, but will develop them, and help you to understand the potential which effective communication skills offer to each consultation.

Ways of communicating

The way in which we most commonly communicate with each other is by talking. We receive information by listening. However, this is by no means the whole story: sometimes the look on a person's face or their posture gives another message to the viewer. Body language or non-verbal communication is an essential part of each interpersonal interaction which we make. Unfortunately, these clues are often very subtle and require skill in elucidation. This section will give you some theories of communication, both verbal and non-verbal.

Verbal communication

There are certain assumptions which we all make about everyday conversations: in most cases only one person speaks at a time; you both stick to the subject being discussed; and there are not prolonged silences.

In professional encounters some of these rules may be changed in order to cover other expectations, which both patient and professional have of the consultation. For example, a professional is deemed to be an expert, so more talking may be expected from the expert (by both participants). Other examples include the use of questions, the use of silences and the role of the professional as an active listener.

There are unwritten rules of speech which we use unwittingly. Some of the functions of these codes which we use in everyday language are set out in Table 3.1, together with examples of their use and what the language denotes. Think of a recent conversation, perhaps with a patient, and analyse it with the help of Table 3.1.

It is possible to see that speech contains both overt and hidden meanings. It is used not only to convey a message but, at times, also to provoke a particular response or behaviour. Later in this chapter we discuss assertiveness, which is also relevant to the use of speech and manipulation of responses. Of course, there are other factors which influence what we express, such as our self-awareness and self-control. As well as being aware of what constrains or develops our own verbal responses, it is important to understand that others have constraints too. The way in which these theories affect our verbal consultation techniques will be discussed later.

Non-verbal communication

It is not uncommon for someone's facial expression or stance to give away what they mean to say, even though the words they use are conveying another meaning. It is even possible to get a message when there are no words exchanged. This is the power of non-verbal communication (NVC).

There are unwritten rules of NVC just as there are with speech. For example, Western people often do not look at each other when speaking, but do when listening. Afro-Caribbeans show the opposite characteristics. Such rules of NVC pertain to personal space, appearance, touch and gestures, as well as facial expression. Some of these rules will be discussed here, but we also recommend that you read one of the books from the reading list at the end of this chapter for a fuller discussion.

The forms and uses of NVC include the following: (1) facial expression; (2) bodily posture and movement; (3) personal appearance; (4) bodily contact or touching; and (5) personal space.

Table 3.1 Codes of speech (from Kagan et al. 1986).

Function	Denotes	Examples
Identified member of social group	Shared knowledge roles	N: I'll get the sphyg and do a BP (jargon) D: And the thyroid antibody titre was 1:26.784932 (imagine! talking shop)
Showing status reflecting interest in the other	Interpersonal attitudes, perceived status roles in a team	N: (on 'phone) Hello Dr. Brown this is Betty (formal/informal address) P: So then I said to Jim (that's Professor Smith, you know—he lives next door to me . . . (one-upmanship, name dropping)
Personal identity	Attitudes, values, character	N: I really like going out to the pub (self disclosure) P: I went to America recently (personal anecdote)
Manipulation or control	Regulation of other's speech	N: How often does the pain come? (closed question—limited reply opportunities) N: Tell me about the pain (open question—many reply opportunities) D: Mm, go on . . . (encouraging) N: So you feel sad (reflecting)
Manipulation and control	Regulation of other's behaviour	N: Take these three times a day (command) D: May I take your blood pressure? (request) N: It's quite normal to feel that way (reassurance)
Informing others, acting in a role	Expertise role	N: You should take these tablets regularly . . . (information) Receptionist: Yes, you are next (answers requests)
Acquiring information/learning	Need for information	P: What's an IVP? (needs explanation) N: Have you had your blood pressure checked before? (needs information)
Expressing emotional state or personal identity	Disturbance, need to convey feelings	P: I hate waiting in that waiting room! (expressing) N: It's bloody ridiculous (swearing, frustrated) Woman: Hello darling! (expressing affection)
Escaping from difficult situations	Unwillingness to face emotions (self or others)	P: Is it cancer? N: Only the doctor can give this information (blocking) N: That didn't hurt, did it? (leading question) P: I'll say hello to St. Peter at the Pearly Gate for you (false reassurance, joking)
Giving facts	Information giving	N: The towel needs replacing (statement) D: Mrs. B. seems brighter today (statement)

D = doctor; N = nurse; P = patient.

1 *Facial expression.* The way the face is configured can denote:

- happiness;
- sadness;
- anger;
- surprise;
- disbelief;
- fear;
- disgust;
- interest.

It is more difficult to tell what people are really feeling if they are smiling. Otherwise, it is usually possible to discriminate between these facial expressions. Facial expressions tend to confirm our emotions, though sometimes the face belies the speech. In consultations it is obviously important to recognize these conflicting occasions, and then attempt to find the real problem.

2 *Bodily posture and movement.* The way we stand, sit or gesture may give away much of how we feel. Someone who is tense and apprehensive may sit in a closed, tight position; for example, arms and legs crossed, shoulders drawn in and hunched up. The opposite is an open, welcoming position, sitting in a relaxed way, arms loose and legs relaxed. Someone who feels superior may sit with feet on a desk, arms behind head, chair pushed back. Most gestures or postures also express a feeling. Can you say what the gestures in Figure 3.1 mean? Gestures and posture are not always this obvious in their meaning, but may be variations on these themes.

3 *Personal appearance.* The way people dress denotes something about themselves. Argyle (1983) said 'The information that is conveyed [by dress] includes social status, occupation, attractiveness, attitudes to other people, like rebelliousness or conformity, and other aspects of personality'.

Some examples of this are easy to identify: Hell's Angels all wear a similar 'uniform' as did punks in their day. Fashion often dictates our appearance; equally important is not following fashion. Many older people wear their best clothes to visit the doctor or nurse. What does this denote?

4 *Bodily contact/touching.* The British are not renowned for touching each other, even in very conventional ways like shaking hands. In France, if one male joins a group of friends, he shakes hands with all the men and kisses the women on both cheeks. Women often kiss all the group. This may happen if the group see each other frequently and if they are young. In Britain, this is a less commonly accepted form of

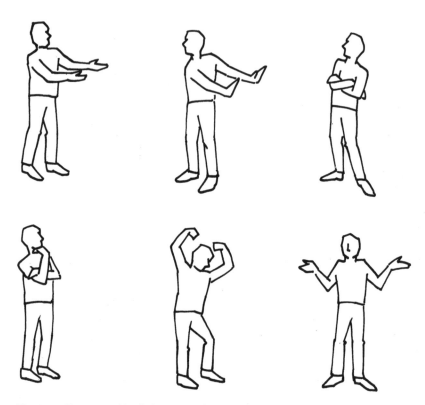

Fig. 3.1 Postures with obvious meanings.

behaviour. For example, it is uncommon for a British nurse or doctor to shake hands with a patient at the beginning of a consultation.

Touch can in itself be therapeutic and some studies have shown that people recover faster if touched by nurses (Argyle 1983).

5 *Personal space.* The distance we put between ourselves and others is affected by our culture and our feelings about the other person. It is now common to think of the desk as a barrier between professional and patient, which distances them and gives the professional power.

Often, as health professionals, we invade a person's territory by examining them and getting closer to them than we would in normal social circumstances. This can be threatening to some people and is a powerful primitive signal of dominance.

If we are to consider people as partners in health care, our NVC must reflect this feeling. Hence, asking permission of people before we invade their territory, and ensuring they sit next to, not opposite, the health carer, are important principles.

The place of health care in individual lives

Concepts of health and illness vary from individual to individual. Some describe themselves as healthy simply when they do not have obvious disease. Others feel healthy only when they are physically and mentally fit. In a world of increasing consumerism with high expectations, most health professionals and consumers would accept the WHO (World Health Organization) definition of health which involves psychological and social well-being and not merely an absence of disease.

There may be many occasions when the pressure of work makes you think that the whole population is feeling unhealthy and are bringing their problems to the surgery. The fact of the matter is that only a small proportion of the symptoms people feel are presented to health care workers at all. Probably 90% of symptoms are coped with without reference. So why do some people bring their symptoms to us and others manage the same symptoms in a different way? The reason is because people have different concepts of health and illness. They have their own 'health understanding' (Pendleton 1981).

This health understanding is made up of a patient's belief about their symptoms, their previous experience of both illness and remedies, and their general attitudes. This understanding might be influenced by factual material or misconception, myth, irrational belief and fear. There has been a lot of research both in the UK (Pendleton 1981; King 1982) and the USA (Becker 1979) which demonstrates that health understanding plays a very important part in why people seek medical advice to start with, and whether they follow the advice that they are given. There are five aspects of the health belief model as described by Becker (1979).

1   Perceived vulnerability—'How likely am I to get that particular problem?'
2   Perceived seriousness—'How serious would the problems be for me?'
3   Perceived cost/benefit of treatment—'What are the pros and cons of having the problem treated?'
4   Cues to action—prompts that people have, such as a TV programme, visit to the surgery or discussion with a friend.
5   Health motivation—the fact that different people have different interests in their health and different motivations to look after it.

This last aspect, health motivation, is made up like health understanding from many sources, such as their experiences or their upbringing. Another factor in personality which affects motivation is 'locus of control', that is where patients think the control of their lives lie. This has been studied in respect to health (Wallston & Wallston 1978) and it was found that the internal controllers, or those people who felt that their future health was a result of their present actions, were more likely to follow medical advice. External controllers, or those people who felt that they had little control over their lives and their health, are much more likely to continue with unhealthy lifestyles and leave the future to chance.

Health understanding and concepts of how health is controlled are very important determinants as to whether patients will follow advice. These two factors are changeable and a skilful health professional can help their patients towards more positive health beliefs with a wish to control their own health. This requires confident communication skills.

Tasks for the consultation

We have put together a series of tasks, based on the work of the Wycombe Primary Care Prevention Project (Havelock *et al.* 1989), that take into consideration the important theoretical background to people's perception of their health and why they then attend the nurse or doctor. The tasks for every consultation are:

- exploration of the problems;
- explanation, negotiation and management planning;
- support and relationship building.

Task 1: Exploration of the problem

This, the first aspect of the nurse – patient consultation, is the basis of all the rest: Why is this person here? What do they want? What do they need? Part of this task is the taking of a traditional history. What are the patient's symptoms and the relationship of those symptoms: where, when, start, finish, made worse, made better, goes where, comes from? This process needs the skilful use of questioning and listening, although a lot of the information needed for this are facts. Often the best way of getting the required information is using an open question and then waiting for the reply.

Patient:	I have a pain in my chest.
Nurse:	Tell me about it (sits back, looks the patient in the eye and smiles).
Patient:	Well it started . . . , goes down my arm . . .
Nurse:	Go on . . .
Patient:	Made worse when I walk, or dig the garden.

Toward the end of this interaction the nurse will probably want to clarify some of the information that she has gained and might use direct or closed questions.

Nurse:	You said the pain came on when you walked, how far before it comes on?
Patient:	About 150 yards.
Nurse:	Is that on the flat or uphill?
Patient:	On the flat. It is shorter going uphill or if I hurry.
Nurse:	What do you do when it comes on?
Patient:	Stop and it goes off . . .

There might also be a need for specific information in other areas and these can be explored in the same way, hopefully with an explanation to the patient.

Nurse:	I would now like to ask you some questions dealing with your general health. Is that OK?
Patient:	Yes.
Nurse:	Do you have any trouble breathing or a cough?
Patient:	No.
Nurse:	Any trouble with your stomach, bowels, etc?

This history-taking also includes gathering information about aspects of the patient's lifestyle that might affect their health—their smoking, drinking, eating and exercise habits. It might also include their previous medical condition and social circumstances. These can be asked about in the same way with a variety of questioning and listening skills.

The second and equally important aspect of exploration of the problem is to explore the patient's health understanding. What they believe, think, understand, and feel about their problem plays a major part in their response to ill health and whether they will follow any advice from the nurse. Exploring the patient's ideas and concerns is a fruitful but sometimes difficult task which needs a sensitive and skilful approach. Some of the skills needed are briefly described here, but further reading in this field would be helpful (such as Pendleton *et al.* 1984 or Neighbour 1988).

Sometimes a straightforward open question can help the patient express his or her fears.

Nurse:	What ideas do you have about what might have caused the pain?

But this question can sometimes produce the reply:

Patient: I don't know, that's why I came to you.

There is obviously a need to sometimes couch the question in a more productive way. Choose one or two that suit you and try them out.

Nurse:	I was having a number of thoughts as you spoke; what were your thoughts?
Nurse:	I would like to find out what you think may be going on—can you put this into words?
Nurse:	Some people might be concerned about having this pain—are you?
Nurse:	I had a patient once who had similar pain and she was very concerned that it was her heart—are you?
Nurse:	Can you tell me what your family's/friends' worries are about the pain?

When the patient is talking more easily about their thoughts and concerns it is possible to be more specific in your questioning and to explore health beliefs, particularly in regard to personal risk factors, such as smoking.

Nurse:	What do you feel are the risks of smoking to you?
Nurse:	What for you are the benefits and costs of stopping smoking?
Nurse:	How might you start to give up?
Nurse:	How can I help you to give up?

The last component in exploration of the problem is a relevant physical examination. The examination is important in most consultations because of the following.

1 It can provide extra information in order to contribute to a management plan.
2 It is expected, in many instances, by the patient.
3 It provides an opportunity to touch the patient which can enhance the relationship.

Examination skills are important but are outside the scope of this chapter. Some are included in the relevant chapters on clinical conditions.

Task 2: Explanation and negotiation

Having decided what the problem is, nurse and patient must reach a decision about further treatment or follow-up. If the person is to be included as a partner in the consultation, then certain processes are essential.

1 The patient must understand the nature of the complaint.
2 Any recommended treatment or follow-up must be clearly understood.
3 The purpose of a need for medication must be understood.
4 The nurse should understand and appreciate how the patient feels, and what they know about their condition.

Presenting information

Anything which a patient is told must be in language which is understood. This is self-evident, but not always practised. Earlier in this chapter codes of speech were discussed, and the way in which using jargon marks out the user as a member of a certain group. Jargon abounds in health care, and it is easy to forget that it is not always understood by the layman. Present information which is either in layman terms, or use the technical term and then fully explain it.

Often the best way is to find out first what the patient believes is the problem, what is believed to be the cause and what they would like to be done.

Nurse:	What do you think caused this? What do you think is the problem?

Provided you ask in a neutral and supportive way, the information will be forthcoming. Once you understand what the patient's beliefs are, you are in a position to identify any accurate knowledge and to build on what the person does know with the relevant correct information.

The patient will not remember all of what you say, so write down anything important to be taken away or use leaflets for this. People generally remember two out of six statements at any one time, and are more likely to retain the early ones. This can be a major problem because people will remember the diagnosis information which comes before the management or self-instruction. One way to alleviate this problem is by structuring information so it is easy to recall. Let the patient know in advance what you are going to talk about:

Nurse:	First I'm going to tell you about your blood pressure level, then about something which might help to control it.

Another way to assist recall is to be specific. General statements like 'take more exercise' are not helpful and more forgettable. Specific recommendations such as 'walk briskly for half an hour each day' are more memorable and attainable.

Having presented the information, ask what the patient thinks about it: Is it understood? Are there any questions? If you are giving information about lifestyle changes, which nurses often do, do they seem feasible? We are now into the business of negotiation.

Negotiation or making plans

Deciding on a recall date might go like this:

Nurse:	Can you come back in three months?
Patient:	No.
Nurse:	When would you like to come back then?
Patient:	In one month—I'd like to be checked up then.
Nurse:	OK. Let's do that.

This is real negotiation. The question which the nurse asked first was intended as a real question. Therefore when the patient was able to express concerns that would be met by an earlier review an amicable solution was negotiated. Listen actively to answers. You must pick out the hidden meanings from what is said overtly. You must be aware of these in negotiations. Be sensitive to underlying fears or concerns, often conveyed by non-verbal communication. Whatever message you are trying to convey will be blocked if the recipient has other things on their mind.

If you are not letting the patient participate in the negotiation, any plans you think you have made may fail. Lifestyle changes are particularly difficult to negotiate because they are often a reflection of other aspects of life. Changing eating habits may affect a whole family or giving up smoking may change the person's image with their workmates. You need all this information to facilitate any changes. No matter how foolish it may sometimes seem to you, it is vital to negotiate.

Persuasion

Sometimes, however, the message is so vital that it requires persuasion. Can you be persuasive? Knowledge does not always change people's behaviour, because behaviour is also affected by beliefs and attitudes. If someone believes that fate influences what is going to happen, then they may see little point in changing their behaviour. Try to understand attitudes and beliefs and base any persuasive message on them.

Being non-judgemental, accepting the patient as they see themselves, will allow them to be honest with you and explore their own beliefs. Furthermore, it is important that you understand your own beliefs and attitudes as well as your communications skills. Are you aware of yourself?

The patient must believe that you are there to help and that you want to help. Warmth in word and posture (looking relaxed, ready to listen) will convey your wish to help. Be confident in your message, know your subject. This will give you credibility and you will be believed.

Certain practical factors will affect the receptiveness of patients. Is your consultation room quiet, is it well lit with chairs placed to facilitate eye contact, and without barriers? Can anyone outside hear what is said? Disruptions detract from concentration, so make sure that you will not be interrupted. Table 3.2 is a checklist for persuasive communication, taken from Coutts and Hardy (1983).

Table 3.2   Checklist for persuasive communication (from Coutts & Hardy 1983).

Do	Do not
Establish a trusting relationship	Be glib
Allow the patient the freedom to participate	Make premature judgements
Be helpful	Be opinionated
Set up a conducive atmosphere	Belittle
Regard the information as confidential	Change the subject

Task 3: The helping relationship

Building a relationship with a patient which is helpful to him or her is central to the aims of nursing (and other) consultations. This section analyses what skills are needed to be helpful. Some of the skills are hard to acquire, partly because they are difficult to measure. They are, however, vital to a helping relationship, and so the following tips are offered for developing them.

Empathy

Empathy has been described as the ability to experience another person's world as if it were one's own without ever losing that 'as if' quality (Murgatroyd 1985). It involves the ability to theorize how someone else is feeling. A way of showing empathy is by attempting to summarize how you imagine a person is feeling and reflecting that back to them.

> Patient: I'll never be able to lose weight. I really hate diets and even when I stick to them I don't lose weight. I've got my job and my family to contend with, you know. It's all such a strain.
>
> Nurse: You sound as though there are many things for you to feel anxious about.
>
> Patient: (*Crying*) Yes I do, I really do, I'm such a failure . . .

In a similar way, content can be reflected for clarification, or to prompt further discussion.

> Patient: These tablets make me feel sick. I'm sure I don't take them regularly you know, so I suppose that's the reason my blood pressure is up?
>
> Nurse: You're saying that you don't take your tablets because they make you feel sick?
>
> Patient: Yes—well, I think they do, but I've always felt sick easily and I think the other tablets suited me better.

Sometimes disclosing something about ourselves can help to establish that we understand how someone feels. It also shows trust. However, such occasions have to be handled with sensitivity or the nurse becomes the focus of the consultation, rather than her patient. Here is an example of self-disclosure.

> Patient: I've got six children and there never seems time for myself.
>
> Nurse: Yes, I understand because I find that having only two children as well as this job is hard-going. I appreciate your feelings.
>
> Patient: Well, you understand then—so what do you think I can do?

Warmth

Showing warmth is not necessarily easy, especially if you do not particularly like the person. You are there to learn from each other—you are seeking their respect and acceptance. Exercise the power of being a helper consciously, having careful regard for its impact on others. The importance of warmth is that it creates a climate within which change can take place.

Be specific and genuine

Being specific is helpful because it narrows down a problem to its component parts, or it pinpoints a feeling. As the helper you are able to be more objective than the patient, and can therefore help to identify specific feelings or problems.

It is hard to teach anyone to be genuine, yet genuineness encourages others to be open about their own feelings. It is clearly not helpful for others to be at the mercy of our daily mood swings and irritability, but genuineness does not mean this. It means being able to occasionally disclose things that we feel will be helpful to another. It requires us to mean what we say. A particularly memorable example of this is a description by Murgatroyd (1985) of a conversation between a nurse and patient who was dying.

> The patient expresses her wish to be put to sleep because she feels so lonely and no-one will care anyhow if she is dead. The nurse reveals that she cares for the patient and will weep for her when she (the patient) dies. This has the effect of giving the woman hope, and lessens her despair.

We do not often encounter such situations in general practice, but sometimes it is right to tell people that they are not alone, or that you feel they are right or wrong. Provided the disclosure is true, and you have considered why you are saying it, it will promote trust and honesty between you and the patient.

Developing helping skills

Although, as we have stated before, it is not easy to acquire helping skills, it is possible to 'work on yourself' to develop your potential. Here are some suggestions which you can do with colleagues, friends and family:

- practice ways of describing feelings;
- enlarge your vocabulary of emotions by looking them up in a dictionary or a thesaurus;
- practice reflecting people's feelings;
- experiment with what you say back to them.

Read about psychology and apply it to yourself and others. Examine your own feelings and emotions: What sort of person are you? Why? Describe yourself to someone you trust. You can say that you want to get some practice. Ask them what they think about your description. When you have the opportunity, describe your thoughts and feelings on a subject to others. Practice self-disclosure.

All these exercises will help you to gain insight into yourself, to understand what makes you tick. This will improve the way in which you can help others to understand themselves.

Nurses often help people to cope with situations that, for one reason or another, are stressful. There are different ways of helping people to cope effectively; Murgatroyd (1985) has made a model of these methods.

1   Help the person face up to the crisis he or she is having. This means encouraging him or her to identify the crisis, the reasons for it and the part he or she is playing in it.
2   Identify, within the crisis, parts of it which can be tackled one at a time. This makes the task less daunting and gives hope of success.
3   Encourage the person to be objective, and not to cloud issues with overwhelming emotion, which makes it impossible to identify solutions.
4   Do not give false reassurances. This is something that is tempting for nurses. It is easy to say 'I am sure everything will be alright' when, in fact, you have no evidence of this.
5   Encourage people to help themselves by identifying with them ways that they can do so. This may be by finding a support amongst family or friends.

Once you have rapport with the patient, you are able to be a helper in a crisis. You will develop rapport by showing empathy, warmth and genuineness, and by being sensitive to all the verbal and non-verbal clues which you are given. In many ways this helping relationship is at the heart of nursing, and underpins this book.

Feeling good about yourself

It is not always easy in a job, which is at times emotionally demanding, to feel that you are coping. How do you learn to feel good about yourself, even when you are wrong or under pressure? Because people are so different from each other, it is not possible to give you a checklist of what to do, but here are some suggestions for you to consider.

Assertiveness

Being assertive means being able to say what you mean, what you want and how you feel in plain language, without feeling the need to soften the blow. It does not mean being aggressive, selfish or manipulative.

Practise saying exactly what you mean in any situation. If you are feeling that you have had an unfair share of the workload say: 'I am feeling that I have been expected to do more than my fair share of the work today and

I would like us to think about how we might change that'. Notice that you are speaking in the first person, rather than saying, for example: 'You have given me too much work'.

The purpose of assertiveness is not to manipulate or blame, but to state a problem and negotiate a solution. You can resist being manipulated yourself by first identifying when it happens and then dealing with it by refusing to be manipulated. An example of manipulation sometimes used at work is: 'I don't understand why you have to take so long with each person, all the rest of us make do with a five-minute consultation, why can't you?'

This is an attempt to manipulate by guilt. The assertive response is: 'I can see that you find this irritating (acknowledging the problem) but I don't understand why I can't have longer appointments if I work longer hours. Is there a problem about doing that?'

There are many techniques which can be used so that you become more assertive. This chapter cannot possibly cover all of them and can only give you a glimpse of what it is all about. Perhaps your first assertive act should be to ask to go on an assertiveness training course. If you cannot do that, get one of the recommended books on the subject.

Your own health

Do you look after your health? Have you been screened lately? Why not? To be fit to carry out your tiring and demanding job, you must pay attention to your own health. If you feel unable to motivate yourself to do this, join a gym, go to a health club or spend a weekend at a health farm. You deserve it, and you will begin to take an interest in your own health.

What do you do about stress? Is there anyone you can talk to about work? Do you exercise regularly to control your stress? Do you make time for yourself, no matter how busy you are? Try to treat yourself, you deserve it.

Sometimes it helps to have a 'mentor' to talk over problems, to help you to cope and to help you pick up signs of stress in yourself. It does not have to be a professional person, a friend or colleague will be just as helpful. You may like to help each other in this way.

One word of advice: is your doctor in the practice you work for? If so, can you get the attention or empathy that you need? Consider seeking another general practitioner. Ask your employer for help in finding one. It is more important that your health is good than that you may offend somebody.

Getting what you deserve

You may have noticed the phrase, 'you deserve it'; it has been used deliberately. Something that will help you feel good is refusing to be a victim or martyr. Many of us are conditioned from our early years to be both, particularly if we are women. The myths are that women must sacrifice themselves for husband, children, parents, pets, the local cricket team and the parent/teacher association, to name but a few. To do so is 'good' and worthy.

There is no great rule that says this should be so. People deserve to have the right to make choices, including choosing not to do something and to take leisure instead. You do deserve free time, space to develop and grow, and to organize your work and play so that you can function at your best. Health is for everyone, and that includes you.

Good consulting needs good practice management

All through this chapter we have been encouraging the nurse – patient contact to be of maximum effectiveness for both partners. It takes a great deal of sensitivity, skill and intense concentration to recognize all the signs from the patient and to portray yourself as you would wish to. All this can be easily scuttled by poor practice management around you. The list shown in Table 3.3 is by no means exhaustive and we are sure that you can add many more examples to it from your own experience.

This chapter emphasizes that a lot of the control of your job is in your hands. How you feel about yourself needs managing as sensitively and skilfully as does the nurse – patient relationship. When you feel good about yourself it helps you feel good about others. However, it needs working on.

Table 3.3 Poor practice management that affects consultations.

1   Interruptions:

Telephone:
  patients wanting advice
  doctors referring patients
  hospitals with results
  receptionists with queries
  wrong numbers

People:
  patients walking in uninvited
  doctors wanting equipment
  health visitors wanting vaccines from the fridge
  receptionists wanting health education booklets
  secretaries wanting milk from the fridge to make coffee

2   Space:
  having to share a room and thus having to rush
  not enough storage space
  poor design of room

3   Equipment:
  no equipment
  wrong equipment
  broken equipment

4   Records:
  wrong records
  jumbled records
  illegible records
  no records
  poorly designed records

5   Booking system:
  no booking system
  too frequent bookings
  double bookings
  too long surgeries
  inappropriate bookings

References

Argyle, M. (1983) *The Psychology of Interpersonal Behaviour*. Penguin, West Drayton.

Becker, M. H. (1979) Understanding patient compliance: the contributions of attitude and other psycho-social factors. In *New Directions in Patient Compliance*, (ed S. Cohen). Lexington Books, New York.

Coutts, L. & Hardy, L. (1983) *Teaching for Health. The Nurse as Health Educator*. Churchill Livingstone, Edinburgh.

Havelock, P. B., Blakeway-Phillips, C. & Schofield, T. P. C. (1989) A co-ordinated card and guidelines for health checks in general practice. (In press.)

Kagan, C., Evans, J. & Kay, B. (1986) *A Manual of Interpersonal Skills for Nurses. An Experimental Approach*. Harper & Row, London.

King, J. B. (1982) *Attributions, Health Beliefs and Health Behaviour*. Doctoral dissertation, University of Oxford, Oxford.

Murgatroyd, S. (1985) *Counselling and Helping*. Methuen and the British Psychological Society, London.

Pendleton, D. (1981) *Doctor Patient Communication*. Doctoral dissertation, University of Oxford, Oxford.

Wallston, R. A. & Wallston, B. S. (1978) *Locus of control and health: a review of the literature*. Health Education Monograph 6, 107 – 117.

Further reading

Dyer, W. (1978) *Pulling Your Own Strings and Our Erroneous Zones*. Avon Self Help, New York. ·

Fast, J. (1978) *Body Language*. Pan Books, London.

Hannay, D. R. (1979) *The Symptom Iceberg*. Routledge & Kegan, London.

Neighbour, R. (1988) *The Inner Consultation*. MTP Press, Lancaster.

Pendleton, D., Schofield, T., Tate, P. & Havelock, P. B. (1984) *The Consultation: An Approach to Learning and Teaching*. Oxford University Press, Oxford.

Peplau, H. (1988) *Interpersonal Relations in Nursing*. Macmillan, London.

Seedhouse, D. & Cribb, A. (1989) *Changing Ideas in Health Care*. J. Wiley & Sons, Chichester.

Tudor Hart, J. & Stilwell, B. (1988) *Prevention of Coronary Heart Disease and Stroke. A Workbook for Primary Health Care Teams*. J. Wiley & Sons, Chichester.

4 Health Education and the Oxford Prevention of Heart Attack and Stroke Project

THERE have been many recent reports and publications (Royal College of General Physicians 1981; Health Education Authority 1984) indicating the growth of interest in and commitment to health promotion and preventive medicine. More general practitioners are extending the systematic and successful approaches to screening, that have paid such dividends in reducing the infant mortality rates and congenital abnormalities, to include the middle-aged and elderly groups. The same enthusiasm and commitment that has been devoted to cervical cytology, for example, now needs to be applied to the prevention of arterial disease. The clinical theme for this chapter is therefore the avoidance of cardiovascular disease.

Much of the expansion of this work has been possible by involving the team, the practice nurse, the health visitor and the district nurse. Practice managers and reception staff have also been crucial in this development by their attention to detail when devising reliable recall methods for both manual and computerized systems. However, there is still a shortfall in the uptake of the Family Practitioner Committee (FPC) reimbursement scheme for ancillary staff, with a national average of only 1.2 staff per general practitioner. In Oxfordshire, where the average is 1.6, it has been calculated that 164 half-time practice nurses, practice managers or reception staff could be employed within the reimbursable levels tomorrow. An inevitable question is, therefore, with more staff, how much more could be achieved? Furthermore, how effective are general practice teams in helping people to change?

Screening and educating for health in general practice

Traditionally, most clinics in general practice, even Well Woman clinics, have been specific-disease-orientated, with such foci as hypertension, diabetes or cervical cancer. They have been mainly designed to facilitate the management of established chronic disease. Probably their most important benefits have been improved practice administration and better record keeping.

Screening well people for risk factors is a different process. It operates without a disease focus. It involves health education, since people are encouraged to appreciate how much more healthy they could be if they altered less healthy aspects of lifestyles. In screening clinics, people attending do not carry a disease label. They are patients only in so far as their names appear on the doctor's list. They are not patients in the illness model since they have no overt symptoms and are not requesting treatment. Health visitors have acknowledged this fact by referring to those with whom they work as clients. Looking at prevention from a well person's viewpoint is quite a change for many staff in general practice. It marks the beginning of planned anticipatory care (Hart 1986).

Lifestyle is not really a medical issue. This is perhaps one of the major factors which leads many nurses and general practitioners to question their right to intervene in their patients' habits and way of life. However, Wallace *et al.* (1987) showed that people do expect their doctors to be concerned about their lifestyle. Furthermore, there is wide public acceptance of the link between lifestyle and health. The dilemma for many people is not whether they should alter their lifestyle, but how.

Although lifestyle itself is not principally a medical issue, the effects of it certainly can be. Reducing disease risk often implies a change in lifestyle. Unfortunately, ambivalence amongst health workers about their ability to change peoples' habits is widespread. Two factors are worth considering.

1　Health professionals have been telling people to give up smoking for many years, however, one-third of the population still indulges. This does not mean that the message to stop smoking is wrong, but it does suggest that we need to develop more effective means of communicating that message. Professionals do not in the end change habits, people do. Communication is a two-way process which involves listening to and learning from the client, as well as imparting information. Much of this is discussed in Chapter 3. Grant, and others, develop this theme in *Coronary Heart Disease: Reducing the Risk* (Grant 1986), a self-study course designed for primary health care team members: doctors, nurses, practice managers and others. It is highly recommended to any practice considering setting up health screening services.

2　Health professionals may be more credible sources of health education than they believe. Russell *et al.* (1979) showed that advice from a general practitioner, backed up by suitable literature, was effective in helping about five per cent of their smokers to give up. Other studies have confirmed this benefit and suggest an even better success rate with Nicorette chewing gum if it is used with minimal professional support (Raw 1986). Intensive stop-smoking group methods cannot claim any better rate.

It may be that a nurse who believes she can motivate people to change can achieve more than one who has no such confidence. Studies are currently under way to examine nurses' effectiveness as health educators, and to study the processes they use.

Requirements for anticipatory care and prevention

The principal requirements for establishing health promotion and prevention will now be discussed. The practical example used in this chapter is targeting prevention of coronary heart disease and it is used to illustrate the points that are made. The examples appear in the tinted boxes.

Setting priorities

Approximately 1 million patients consult their local health centre or surgery every weekday. Many of these will fall into groups with screenable risks. Before structuring this health prevention effectively, priorities for screening have to be set. Wilson, in his criteria for screening, set the following guidelines.

1 The condition screened for should be an important one.
2 There should be an acceptable treatment for patients with the disease.
3 The facilities for diagnosis and treatment should be available.
4 There should be a recognized latent or early symptomatic stage.
5 The test or examination should be acceptable to the population.
6 The cost (including diagnosis and subsequent treatment) should be economically balanced in relation to expenditure on medical care as a whole.

> The Office of Population, Censuses and Surveys (OPCS) provides data on the most common disease mortalities. In Oxfordshire, as in the rest of Britain, ischaemic heart disease is the top killer, as shown in Figure 4.1. This strongly demonstrates the need to screen for high blood pressure and the need to counsel about smoking and diet.

Protected time

Protected time must be allocated for screening clinics, or time dedicted to screening during the normal treatment room duties. In the ideal world, sufficient time should be allowed to see the requisite number of patients to ensure that all the population are screened within an agreed timetable

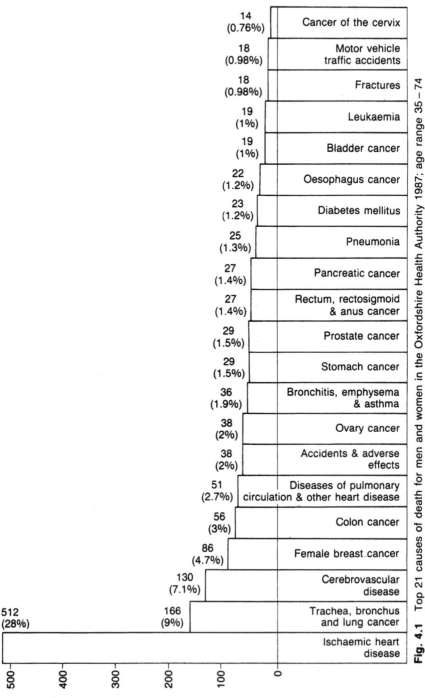

Fig. 4.1 Top 21 causes of death for men and women in the Oxfordshire Health Authority 1987; age range 35–74 (Office of Population, Censuses and Surveys 1987).

(Table 4.1). Extra consultation time (i.e. 20 minutes) is needed because so much of health teaching is concerned with behavioural change. This tests the educational and communication abilities of the nurse. The nurse should consider the list below.

1 Find out what beliefs a person holds.
2 Negotiate changes that could be made.
3 Set goals.

Table 4.1 Number of nursing hours needed for a population of 9000.

1 One third of population in 34 – 65 age group = 3000

2 Assume 6 hours dedicated to prevention per week (two clinics 3 – 6 p.m.) with health check every 20 min
   Therefore the theoretical maximum is 18 patients per week
   In reality allow 15 per week, because of tea breaks, 'did not attends' and follow-ups (needing 10 min appointments)

3 15 × 47 weeks (5 weeks annual leave) = 705 patients *or* 3525 patients every 5 years
   This allow for new patients joining practice and the possibility of extending, after 2 or more years, the age group to include the 30 – 34 year olds

   • 90% of the patient population consult every 5 years
   • 8% do not arrive for appointments (in Oxford)
   • 3% decline the invitation (in Oxford)

Coronary heart disease is of such epidemic proportions that the majority of the population need help with reducing the saturated fat content of their diet and encouragement to increase the amount of exercise they take. Smokers, hypertensives and those with a family history of early heart disease must all be identified.

An organized system of recruitment and recall

To achieve individual health education for everyone, the primary health care team can capitalize on the contact between the patient and the health centre or surgery for some other reason, by offering them a health check. Seventy per cent of patients will consult every year and more than 90% consult within 5 years. The benefit of the primary care team is that the self-employed and unemployed, who would otherwise miss out on occupational screening, are routine attenders at the surgery. This method of recruiting is known as the opportunistic method.

Other screening programmes rely on a member of the primary care team selecting everyone in the age group to be screened and sending written invitations. A combination of both methods can be adopted. The advantages and disadvantages of each system are illustrated in Table 4.2.

If it is cancer or coronary heart disease that is to be tackled, then the advantage of opportunistic screening is that high risk patients consult more often. For example, smokers consult twice as often as non-smokers. People in social classes IV and V, in whom coronary heart disease is 2 – 3 times more common, consult more frequently.

Table 4.2   The advantages and disadvantages of different screening methods.

Opportunistic	Formal
Advantages	
Personal face-to-face invitation	Satisfaction of knowing that everyone has been invited
No postal costs	
No danger of writing to patients who have died	Can regulate the flow of patients by listing out a certain number each month
Can reach 90% of patients within 5 years	Protected time is automatically built in to screening clinics
Can work with out-of-date age – sex registers, or with no age – sex register	
Flow can be regulated by the receptionist not asking patients on certain days	
Disadvantages	
Needs systematic method of tagging the notes to ensure that a record is kept of who has been screened	Lower response rate than the face-to-face invitation
Relies on continuous commitment and enthusiasm to invite patients	Cost is higher with postage, stationery and clerical time in searching for the notes and writing invitations
Takes extra (though a small amount) time for the receptionists to invite people in	
Misses at least 10% of patients at the end of 5 years (but these could be offered written invitations at the end of 5 years if record kept of those screened on an age – sex register)	

Resources

The Health Education Authority produces a wide range of leaflets, booklets, posters and other materials designed to help the health educator (nurse or doctor) in their work with the public. This literature is well produced, up-to-date, authoritative and free from commercial bias. It is also free of charge to practices from health promotion units run by the district health authorities.

Unfortunately, a glance around the consulting rooms of many practices will reveal that much of the health promotion material used has been supplied by commercially motivated pharmaceutical companies. There is often nothing wrong with this, but the advice contained may not be compatible with currently accepted recommendations, such as those produced by the National Advisory Committee on Nutritional Education (NACNE) (1983). Charities, like the British Heart Foundation, are also useful sources of health education literature, some of which is free of charge.

Supporting people through change can involve repeat clinic appointments. It might also require the use of other agencies, not all of them professional. Some practice nurses compile directories of suitable local facilities like the Weight Watchers groups, Look After Yourself classes at local colleges, or keep fit groups. Information on these is available from health education units, sports centres, local papers, libraries, churches, volunteer bureaux, local Community Health Councils.

The Oxford Prevention of Heart Attack and Stroke Project

A research project using human 'MOT' checks tested whether it was feasible to identify and recall the middle-aged population of men and women for cardiovascular risk factors. The human MOT is a nickname for a simple health check. The role of a primary care facilitator and a nurse with a primary care background to help the primary health care team, was also tested (Fullard et al. 1987). Help with establishing a clinic can be obtained from the local primary care facilitator, whose list of tasks is covered in Table 4.3.

Table 4.3 Tasks of a facilitator (from Muir Gray 1987).

Act as a cross-pollinator of good ideas from practice to practice

Initiate practice meeting to discuss workload, costs, method of screening, protocols (diagnosis, referral, management, team roles)

Offer help with baseline audit, e.g. blood pressure recording

Assist receptionist and practice manager with methods of identifying patients to be invited and tagging of notes

Guidance of practice nurse/health visitor in screening procedures, e.g. referral of risk factors to general practitioner, revision in blood pressure measurement technique

Provide information and back-up service, e.g. suggest drafts for invitation handout and health summary card, sources of free health education literature, height/weight charts, teaching aids

Encourage assessment of progress, e.g. by repeat audits, log books in nurse clinics

Although the project was based on a design developed for arterial disease prevention, the method could easily be adapted to organize other screening clinics for the young or elderly. This section describes the Oxford Project.

Steps in starting an 'MOT' clinic

Know where you are starting from

A small audit (or record review) of a sample of notes will give the team an estimate of how well they are doing before starting the clinic. A repeat audit may be done in 2.5 years time (halfway to the 5-year target) to assess progress. If blood pressure, smoking habits and weight (or an indication of obesity) are to be measured, then a baseline and progress audit may be prepared by completing using the following details:

1 Record the risk factors detailed in the notes from a sample of men and women aged between 35 and 64 years (100 – 200 records).
2 Check these records for the following and record the percentage of notes which contain these details:

   • blood pressure measurement;
   • smoking habits;
   • weight or indication of obesity;
   • alcohol consumption;
   • did not consult in 5-year period.

The audit, excluding those who did not consult, will indicate the scale of the task facing the practice. Repeat audits measure progress compared to the baseline figures.

The Oxford Project (1986) has produced audit guidelines to help practices to conduct an audit. However, many practices will be within districts in which facilitators are appointed who can provide local support (see Figure 4.2). These may be contacted through the local Health Education Units or the FPC.

Need for extra labour

The extra costs must also be considered, and the cost of employing a practice nurse for 10 hours per week on mid-point of the present (1989 – 90) pay scale is given in Table 4.4.

Table 4.4   Costs of employing a practice nurse (1989 – 90 pay scale).

	Grade F	Grade G	Grade H
Hourly rate	5.92	6.65	7.38
Weekly rate (10 hours)	59.20	66.50	73.80
Less FPC 70% reimbursement	17.60	19.95	22.14
Less tax relief on remaining 30%	10.65	11.97	13.28
Net cost to practice	£10.65	£11.97	£13.28

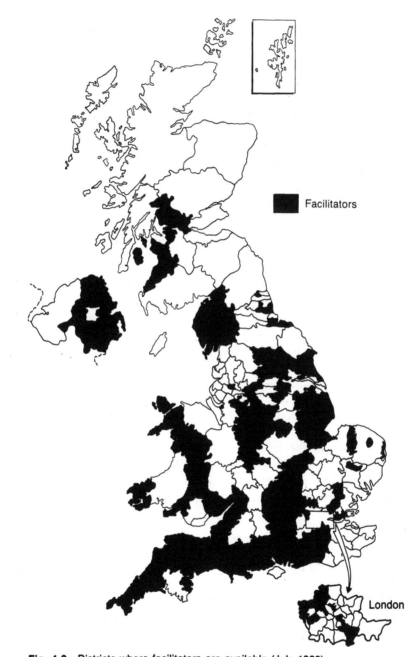

Fig. 4.2 Districts where facilitators are available (July 1989).

Need for extra space

If the middle-aged population are to be screened, then some clinics held outside office hours should be offered to meet the need of the target population. There is, as yet, no evidence that the early morning clinic (8 a.m. – 8.30 a.m), the late evening clinic (5 – 7 p.m.), or the Saturday morning clinic are more or less successful in the number of people attending. The opportunistic method using receptionists resulted in most people (92%) arriving for their appointment.

Equipment checking and training needs

Before embarking on a screening programme for hypertension, it is worthwhile checking to see whether the sphygmomanometers are reading accurately and that an obese-adult-size cuff is available. Several of the pharmaceutical company representatives will service sphygmomanometers and supply alternative adult-size cuffs free of charge. The cuffs may alternatively be purchased at a very modest price. Weighing scales should be matched for accuracy with others in the practice. The beam balance type is the most accurate.

It is essential that the health professional doing the screening is measuring blood pressure in the most accurate way. The local district facilitator may offer hypertension training courses, and he/she will be able to offer an individual session to revise blood pressure measurement. The British Hypertension Society produces guidelines and approves several courses being conducted.

Knowledge about the latest information on nutrition, alcohol and smoking cessation counselling is essential. Doctors and nurses hold such high credibility in the public trust of their advice on health matters, that it behoves everyone to give the most appropriate advice (Francis *et al.* 1989).

Running and evaluating an 'MOT' clinic

Health summary card and protocol

When recording patient details it is advisable to start off with a neutral question, such as family history, rather than asking about smoking, occupation or use of the oral contraceptive pill. Health summary cards are available free from Stuart Pharmaceuticals.* These give guidelines for the nurses to work from, as illustrated in Figure 4.3. Some practices will want to develop their own cards.

*Stuart Pharmaceuticals Ltd, Stuart House, 50 Alderley Road, Wilmslow, Cheshire SK9 1RE.

Name _____

DOB		SMWD		No.	

Own Occupation
Partner's Occupation

Date	Date	Date	
1st B/P	2nd B/P	3rd B/P	Mean if applicable

Weight	Ideal Weight	Height

Nutrition Advice	Exercise

Smoker	Cigarettes	Pipe	Since 19
Non Smoker	Never	Stopped 19	

Family History of CVA or MI

Diabetes	Yes	Insulin	OHD	Diet
	No			

Oral Contraception Years of Use	Current	Past	Never

Last Cervical Smear	Date	Result

Rubella	Immune	Yes	No	Date
	Vaccination	Yes	No	Date

Date of Tetanus	1st	2nd	3rd	Booster

Urine Date	Protein	Sugar

Alcohol

Notes/Advice given/Further action

Fig. 4.3 Health Summary Card.

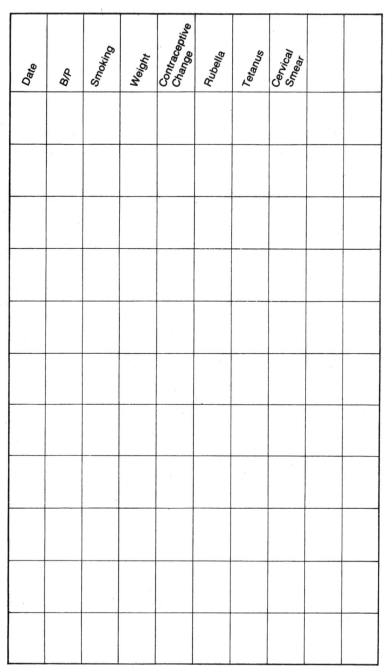

SP4748ap

Fig. 4.3 Health Summary Card *continued*.

The blood pressure protocol was aimed at the 35 – 64 age group and is illustrated in Figure 4.4. The systolic measurement is now considered a better predictor of stroke (Lichtenstein *et al.* 1985), therefore even if the diastolic pressure is less than 90 mmHg where the systolic pressure is raised it is important to recall the patient for an average of three further readings at suitable intervals.

The Oxford Prevention of Heart Attack and Stroke Project team developed a three-way system of recalling patients for mildly raised hypertension to ensure no-one was missed. Firstly, and perhaps most importantly, the patient was advised to put a reminder in a diary that a recheck was due in a year's time. Secondly, the notes were tagged with the month and year the

Checklist before measuring the blood pressure (BP).

1 Patient sitting

2 Note fear/anxiety/anger/cold, if present

3 ? Empty bladder

4 ? Adequate cuff to encircle arm

5 Rate of fall of pressure 2 mmHg per second

6 Record to nearest 2 mmHg

7 Diastolic blood pressure phase V (complete absence of sound) unless this is zero, then use phase IV (muffling) and record 'IV' after recording in medical notes

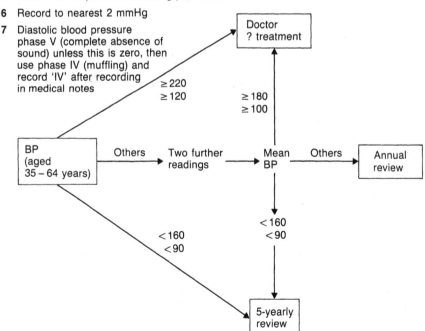

Fig. 4.4 Blood pressure protocol for nurses.

blood pressure check was next due; and thirdly, the patient's name, address, telephone number and level of blood pressure on the third reading were entered in a simple box file held by the nurse. Should the patient not have arrived for the appointment by the end of the month, the nurse then wrote or telephoned the patient. Using this method, 80% of patients were followed up (Mant *et al.* 1989).

No formal protocol was designed for the recall of patients with a weight or smoking problem, but all patients were invited back in approximately 1 month's time to ask about progress. This procedure is based on the results of Jamrozik's study on smoking cessation which indicated that a follow-up appointment increased the cessation rate. Similarly, the study by Kenkre *et al.* (1985) showed that a nurse working in a hypertension clinic succeeded in a 22% cessation rate in their smokers by using the follow-up methods.

The nurses were supplied with lists of local slimming clubs by the local dietitian to capitalize on the community support, exercise classes and leisure facilities available. Similarly, nurses were encouraged to know which supermarkets stocked the low fat, high fibre foods they recommended. Patients had random cholesterol checks if they had either a family history of arterial disease, or had multiple risk factors. If the cholesterol level was raised, then the patient had a full lipid test done.

Evaluating progress

A log book is a simple, cheap way of knowing how many patients the nurse has seen and the risk factors that have been identified. Rewards can be given when the target number has been reached for the month!

A repeat audit of a sample of records might also establish what proportion of women patients have, for example, had a cervical smear within the last 3 or 5 years.

Cervical smear audit: select sample of notes from females aged 35 – 65 years. Exclude hysterectomies from the total number of women. Record the percentage of women with the following details and discuss the results.

1   Had a smear within the last 3 years.
2   Had a smear within the last 4 – 5 years.
3   Had a smear but not within the last 5 years.
4   No trace of ever having had a smear.
5   Refusals.

The audit results after 5 years of the Oxford Prevention of Heart Attack and Stroke Project are displayed in Figure 4.5. These compare the rates in intervention and control practices.

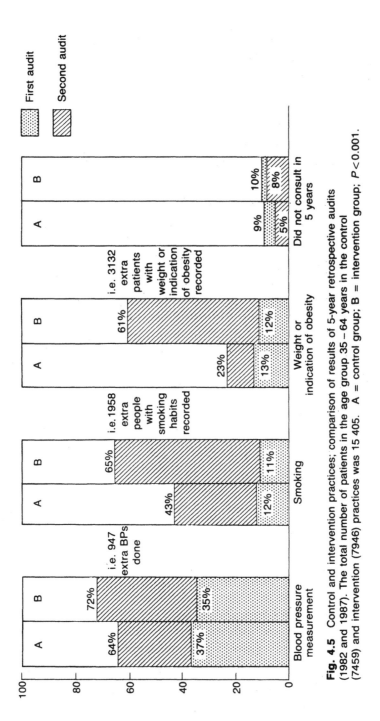

Fig. 4.5 Control and intervention practices; comparison of results of 5-year retrospective audits (1982 and 1987). The total number of patients in the age group 35 – 64 years in the control (7459) and intervention (7946) practices was 15 405. A = control group; B = intervention group; $P < 0.001$.

Key points for MOT clinics

1   Make sure that your screening fulfils the criteria of what is really worth-while doing.
2   Establish a baseline.
3   Adopt a 'whole population' approach but ensure that those in the high risk categories are given extra help and follow-up.
4   Give preventive medicine 'protected time'.
5   Update yourself by extra training, reading and visits to other practices that are screening.
6   Use your local facilitator to help with establishing protocols, introducing the method of screening and establishing methods of recall.
7   Feedback results of the screening clinic to other team members.
8   Evaluate progress by audit to further improve the service you are providing for your patients.

Teamwork

Above all, starting an MOT clinic means that teamwork within the practice can begin to become a reality. The need for professionals to talk to each other, to share knowledge, experience and skills becomes more urgent. Where several people are giving advice on health and lifestyle, consistency is essential, as the Crisp Street Practice (1987) have found. The transition may not be painless. It involves all members of the team accepting that no-one has a monopoly of knowledge, or all the answers.

Marsh and Channing (1988) describe improvements in the preventive health care of a relatively deprived community within their own practice. It is clear from their report that this could not have happened without real teamwork.

The potential for teamwork is there. The benefits for patients, and by implication for the health of the whole population, could be considerable.

References

Crisp Street Practice (1987) Developing a computerised preventive programme. *The Practitioner*, **231**, 1634 – 1639.

Francis, J., Roche, M., Mant, D., Jones, L. & Fullard, E. (1989) Would primary health care workers give appropriate dietary advice after cholesterol screening? *British Medical Journal*, **298**, 1620 – 1622.

Fullard, E. M., Fowler, G. H. & Gray, J. A. M. (1987) Promoting prevention in primary care: controlled trial of low technology, low cost approach. *British Medical Journal*, **294**, 1080 – 1082.

Grant, J. G. (1986) Health promotion skills and the individual patient. In *Coronary Heart Disease: Reducing the Risk*, (ed). Open University Press, Reading.

Hart, J. T. (1986) Coronary heart disease prevention in primary care. In *Coronary Heart Disease: Reducing the Risk*, (ed). Open University Press, Reading.

Health Education Authority (1984) The Canterbury Report. Coronary Heart Disease: a plan for action, interdisciplinary workshop conference, (ed G. Rose). Pitman, London.

Jamrozik, K., Vessey, M., Fowler, G., Wald, N., Parker, G., Vanakis, H. (1989) Controlled trial of three different anti-smoking interventions in general practice. *British Medical Journal*, **298**, 1499 – 1503.

Kenkre, J., Drury, V. W. M. & Lancashire, R. J. (1985) Nurse management of hypertension clinics in general practice assisted by a computer. *Family Practice*, **2**(1), 17 – 22.

Lichtenstein, M. J., Shipley, M. J. & Rose, G. (1985) Systolic and diastolic blood pressures as predictors of coronary heart disease mortality in the Whitehall study. *British Medical Journal*, **291**, 243 – 245.

Mant, D., McKinlay, C., Fuller, A., Randall, T., Fullard, E. & Muir, J. (1989) Three year follow-up of patients with raised blood pressure identified at health checks in general practice. *British Medical Journal*, **298**, 1360 – 1362.

Marsh, G. N. & Channing, D. M. (1988) Narrowing the health gap between a deprived and an endowed community. *British Medical Journal*, **296**, 173 – 176.

National Advisory Committee of Nutritional Education (1983) *A Discussion Paper on Proposals for Nutritional Guidelines for Health Education in Britain*. Health Education Council, London.

Office of Population, Censuses & Surveys (1987).

Oxford Prevention of Heart Attack and Stroke Project Team (1986) *Guidelines for Audits in General Practice*. OPHASP, Oxford.

Raw, M. (1986) Does nicotine chewing gum work? In *Coronary Heart Disease: Reducing the Risk*, (ed). Open University Press, Reading.

Royal College of General Practitioners (1981) *Prevention of Arterial Disease in General Practice*. Report No. 19. RCGP, London.

Russell, M. A. H., Wilson, C., Taylor, C. & Baker, C. D. (1979) Effect of general practitioners' advice against smoking. *British Medical Journal*, ii, 231 – 235.

Wallace, P. G., Brennan, P. J. & Haines, A. P. (1987) Are general practitioners doing enough to promote healthy lifestyle? *British Medical Journal*, **294**, 940 – 942.

Wilson, J. M. G. (1965) *Some principles of early diagnosis and detection*. Office of Health Economics, London.

5 Care of Patients with Asthma

ASTHMA is a very common chronic disease. Approximately 15% of children and 5% of adults suffer from the condition in the United Kingdom. It is frequently under-diagnosed, under-treated and poorly followed-up. Many patients, or parents of asthmatic children, are given insufficient information about the condition. Unfortunately there are still approximately 2000 deaths each year. (On average five people die each day in this country.) Eighty to ninety per cent of these deaths could be avoided by better management and more appropriate treatment of asthma.

Most asthmatics, probably as many as 95%, should be managed in the community. The potential workload for a general practitioner is considerable: a doctor with 2500 patients will have approximately 125 current asthmatics. The challenge of good asthma care lies in the correct diagnosis, treatment and management, as well as patient eduction and planned follow-up. This can be achieved by teamwork between doctors and other health professionals. More practice time needs to be created and this can be achieved by extending the nurse's role.

Anatomy and physiology

In normal breathing, air passes through the nasal cavities where it is warmed, moistened and filtered. It continues through the pharynx and larynx and into the trachea which divides into the right and left bronchi (Figure 5.1).

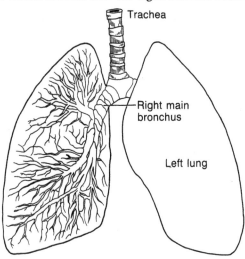

Fig. 5.1 Representational diagram of the lower respiratory tract.

Both the trachea and bronchi contain cartilage in their walls. The bronchi continue to divide and subdivide and these smaller airways, which have now lost their cartilage, are called bronchioles. The bronchioles terminate in clusters of thin-walled sacs called alveoli (Figure 5.2) and it is here, surrounded by a network of capillaries, where the air and blood meet and where the gas exchange takes place.

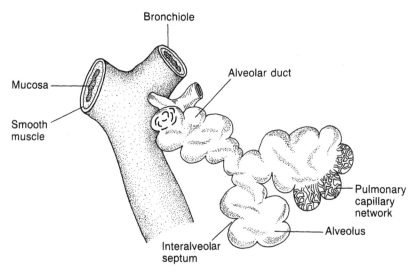

Fig. 5.2   Diagram of the bronchioles and alveoli.

In asthma the airways narrow, resulting in airways obstruction. The bronchial smooth muscle goes into spasm, an excess of mucus is produced, and the bronchial lining and muscle become inflamed and swollen (Figure 5.3).

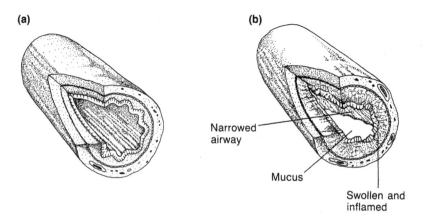

Fig. 5.3   Differences between (a) a normal bronchiole; and (b) an asthmatic bronchiole.

Asthma is not an easy condition to define as it covers a wide range of symptoms which can vary greatly in both severity and frequency. The most straightforward definition is reversible airways obstruction. One of the main features of asthma is over-sensitive airways, known as bronchial hyperreactivity. Asthmatics are more sensitive to inhaled irritants than people without the condition.

Once a diagnosis has been made, it is important to call the condition asthma so the appropriate advice and treatment can be given.

Asthma has been classified into extrinsic and intrinsic types (Table 5.1).

Table 5.1 Differences between extrinsic and intrinsic types of asthma.

Extrinsic	Intrinsic
Starts in childhood	Starts in adulthood
Episodic	Persistent symptoms
Family history of allergy (and strong association with hayfever, allergic rhinitis and eczema)	
Obvious triggers	Often no identifiable triggers other than respiratory tract infection

However, whilst it is of interest to know about the classification of asthma it should not affect the way in which the disease is treated. Many people assume that childhood asthma is curable. Unfortunately this is not so and whilst many children do appear to 'grow out' of it, it has to be remembered that once someone has had asthma, he or she is always potentially asthmatic. A significant proportion of adult asthmatics have asthma in childhood and are then symptom-free for some years, only to find the condition returns in later life. In children, two boys to every one girl have asthma but as the teenage years approach, the numbers even out. After middle age more women than men develop asthma.

Trigger factors

There are many trigger factors which may provoke asthma, which include:

- infection;
- exertion;
- allergy;
- chemical (food, drugs, smoke).

The most common is an upper respiratory tract infection. Exercise, cold air, laughing, coughing and hyperventilation can all trigger attacks.

Allergies to such things as house dust mites, pollens, fungi and pets are common culprits as well as non-specific dusts, fumes and cigarette smoke. Some foods and drinks (such as tartrazine in food colouring, red wine and beer) may set off an attack but this is not very common. Beta-blocking agents, aspirin and non-steroidal anti-inflammatory drugs (NSAIDs) can all precipitate bronchospasm. There is no evidence to suggest that emotion is an underlying cause, although anxiety, anger, depression or stress may bring on an attack in a patient known to have asthma.

Since 1982, occupational asthma has been recognized as an industrial disease and there are specified substances accepted as asthma-inducing for which compensation may be paid.

Symptoms

Asthma certainly has a higher profile these days. Unfortunately, however, there are still many patients whose asthma is unrecognized or undiagnosed, or whose symptoms could be improved dramatically by correct treatment. Many patients, particularly adults, do not consult their doctors either because they have become accustomed to being wheezy or breathless (and think this is normal), or because they know they have a problem but think the doctor cannot do anything for them. A mother with a chesty child is much more likely to consult the doctor early, but still the diagnosis can be missed and an antibiotic too frequently prescribed for a presumed chest infection.

It is important to remember that asthma is due to variable airflow obstruction and very frequently on presentation at the surgery the patient is symptomless, without any demonstrable airways obstruction.

Many patients with asthma can be diagnosed on history alone, but it is very important to enquire about symptoms. The main symptoms of asthma are:

- wheeze;
- shortness of breath (dyspnoea);
- recurrent cough.

These symptoms do not necessarily all occur at the same time and for some patients a cough may be the only symptom. Night-time cough is extremely common in children and many of these will prove to have asthma.

Diagnosis

Peak expiratory flow rate

The diagnosis of asthma can be confirmed (when bronchospasm is occurring) by using the peak flow meter (Figure 5.4, see page 71). This measures the maximum rate of airflow obstruction during expiration and it is expressed in litres per minute. It is important to remember that even though a patient may have a normal peak flow measurement when seen in the surgery, this can change dramatically within a very short time. It is often useful to lend patients a peak flow meter for a few days so they can record their flow during a 24-hour period. This will demonstrate the variability of airflow and will also give the patient some insight into his or her condition.

In children there is little difference in the normal peak expiratory flow rate (PEFR) values between boys and girls. A child of 3′ 9″ (114 cm) would expect to blow about 175 l/min. Normal values for adults are between 400 and 600 l/min (approximately 400 – 500 for women and 600 for men). The measurements will depend on age, sex and height of the patient. Peak flow rates vary in normal subjects, but variations of 20% or more between the lowest and highest readings should confirm the diagnosis of asthma. Many patients with asthma have peak flow readings that are steady during the day, but, due to bronchial hyper-reactivity, have a dramatic drop during the early hours of the morning. This is known as the morning dip. Some may show violent swings in the daytime. This can be due to exposure to triggers or because the asthma therapy has worn off or has not been taken.

Patients with very unstable peak flow measurements are at risk from sudden death especially during the night.

Specific tests using peak flow meters

Reversibility tests

One way of demonstrating reversible airways obstruction is to reverse the obstruction with anti-asthma therapy. The PEFR is measured before and after administering a bronchodilator and a rise of 15 – 20% in PEFR will confirm the diagnosis of asthma. An inhaled β_2-stimulant (e.g. salbutamol, terbutaline) may be used in which case the PEFR should be remeasured after 10 – 15 minutes. Alternatively an inhaled anticholinergic (e.g. ipratropium) may be given when the PEFR should be remeasured 30 – 40 minutes after drug administration.

A steroid trial may be used when there is little or no response to bronchodilator therapy. The usual procedure is to lend the patient a peak flow meter and for about a week, twice daily recordings are taken as a baseline. Oral prednisolone 30 – 40 mg (0.6 mg/kg body weight) is given as a single dose after breakfast each morning for 2 weeks and the PEFR is measured twice daily to assess the response. The steroid trial does not commit the patient to long-term systemic steroid therapy since this is usually replaced with inhaled steroids which are considerably lower in dose.

Exercise test

An exercise test may be used when a patient's history is very suggestive of asthma but the PEFR readings are normal when measured at consultation. The rationale is to provoke bronchoconstriction by taking exercise. The peak flow is measured and then 6 minutes vigorous exercise taken, outside if possible. The PEFR is remeasured on completion of the exercise and then at 5-minute intervals up to and including 15 minutes. The positive exercise test will show a change from initial bronchodilation to bronchoconstriction which is maximal at 3 – 7 minutes. The typical asthmatic will show a drop of greater than 15%. The reaction is usually transient but it can be reversed or prevented with an inhaled β_2-stimulant. It is important to remember that it is not always possible to provoke exercise-induced asthma by carrying out a specific test. Often there is a more satisfactory result if the patient borrows a peak flow meter and records their PEFR when symptoms are apparent during recreational exercise. Cross-country running and sport played during the winter months are particularly troublesome for the exercise-induced asthmatic, whereas swimming in a warm, moist atmosphere rarely causes problems.

Home monitoring

Nowadays many patients are in a position either to buy a peak flow meter or to borrow one from the practice. As yet they are not available on the National Health Service but may be obtained from the National Asthma Campaign headquarters at a reasonable cost. A peak flow meter is better borrowed if required solely to confirm the diagnosis of asthma, but it has also become an essential tool for monitoring the control of known asthmatics. Patients chart their peak flow, if possible 3 – 4 times a day including early in the morning and late evening. It should also be measured at night if they are woken with symptoms.

It is important to educate the patient carefully in how to use the peak flow meter (Figure 5.4).

Beware of the mouth blower—this problem can be identified if it is noticed that the patient puffs out the cheeks when blowing into the meter. These readings will be inaccurate.

Paediatric (low reading) peak flow meters are available with small mouth pieces. Teaching children how to use a peak flow meter may be done in several ways. The most effective is for them to blow out candles. It must be remembered though that it is of more value to teach a small child how to use an inhaler device before attempting peak flow measurement, since this is a more important technique to master.

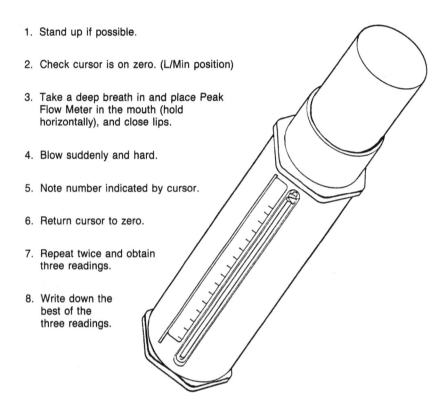

1. Stand up if possible.

2. Check cursor is on zero. (L/Min position)

3. Take a deep breath in and place Peak Flow Meter in the mouth (hold horizontally), and close lips.

4. Blow suddenly and hard.

5. Note number indicated by cursor.

6. Return cursor to zero.

7. Repeat twice and obtain three readings.

8. Write down the best of the three readings.

Fig. 5.4 The Wright mini Peak Flow Meter.

Other diagnostic tests

There are further specialized tests and investigations that may be carried out to confirm the diagnosis of asthma but for the majority of asthmatic patients they are unnecessary. For selected newly diagnosed adult asthmatics, a chest X-ray may be taken to exclude other diseases. Sometimes a blood test for haemoglobin estimation is carried out to rule out anaemia. Skin tests are only rarely done these days, although they may provide further evidence of atopy, they are of no value in the normal management of asthma.

Treatment

There is now a wide range of drugs available to treat asthma. These can be divided broadly into acute (relieving) or prophylactic (preventive) therapies.

Table 5.2   Acute (relieving) and prophylactic (preventive) therapies for asthma treatment.

Acute therapy	Prophylactic therapy
Bronchodilators:	Corticosteroids
β_2-stimulants	Sodium cromoglycate (Intal)
anticholinergics	Nedocromil (Tilade)
methylxanthines (theophyllines)	

Apart from oral corticosteroids and theophyllines, all the drugs listed are best given by inhalation

Bronchodilators

These drugs work by relaxing the contracted bronchial smooth muscle.

Beta$_2$-stimulants

These are the most popular anti-asthma drugs. They act on the sympathetic nervous system to stimulate bronchodilation. Their onset of action is extremely quick. They have a wide margin of safety with few side effects apart from tremor, occasional muscle cramps and tachycardia. They can be used to relieve symptoms due to bronchoconstriction or used prophylactically, especially against exercise-induced asthma. Asthmatics who have only occasional mild symptoms are best managed with β_2-stimulant to be taken as required.

Examples are salbutamol (Ventolin), terbutaline (Bricanyl) or fenoterol (Berotec). The usual dose is two puffs as required, up to 4 – 6 times daily.

Anticholinergic drugs

These inhibit the bronchoconstricting vagus reflex of the parasympathetic nervous system, leading to bronchodilation (i.e. they work against the nerves which constrict the bronchi). Their mode of action is complementary to that of the β_2-stimulants. They have a latent period of about 30 minutes and do not always have an effect so it is sensible to do a reversibility test before using them on a regular basis. They are used mainly in older patients and infants. There are few side effects, the most common being a dry mouth.

The usual dose is two puffs, four times daily. The only drug of importance in this group is ipratropium bromide (Atrovent).

Methylxanthines (theophyllines)

The methylxanthines are a group of drugs which act as bronchodilators in a different way from β_2-stimulants. They have other actions which are not fully understood. Whilst effective against asthma symptoms, they can have toxic effects and the margin of safety is narrow. The long-acting preparations have a place, especially as supplementary therapy for nocturnal and early morning symptoms. Methylxanthines may be used for all age groups but cannot be given by inhalation. The side effects are restlessness, headache, nausea and behavioural problems with children. Care must be taken to avoid over-dosing; indeed, the combination of oral and intravenous preparations is potentially fatal. Since it is important to titrate the right dose against the patient's symptoms, it is frequently necesssary to arrange serum theophylline levels (clotted sample) to achieve maximum dosing but to avoid troublesome or serious side effects.

Examples are theophylline (Nuelin, Slo-phyllin, Uniphyllin) and aminophylline (Phyllocontin). The usual dose is 175 – 225 mg, 1 – 2 tablets twice daily for theophylline and 25 – 30 mg, 1 – 2 tablets twice daily for aminophylline.

Corticosteroids

The mechanism of action of corticosteroids is still not fully understood, but they do exert an anti-inflammatory effect. They reduce mucosal oedema and mucus hypersecretion and are very effective at reducing hyperreactivity.

Systemic steroids

Whilst systemic steroids have been used in the treatment of asthma since the 1950s they are, in general, underused. Their effects are certainly often life-saving and they play an essential role in asthma care. Studies of asthma deaths have regularly shown that the absence of steroid treatment was an important factor. Unfortunately, their long-term use is associated with many side effects such as diabetes, hypertension, Cushing's disease, osteoporosis and peptic ulceration, as well as growth retardation in children. However, whilst they are not without potential problems, short, high-dose courses can be life-saving and this regimen is without important side effects. Approximate doses for acute attacks are 40 – 50 mg for a man, 30 – 40 mg for a woman and 20 – 30 mg for a child. The correct dose can be calculated by giving 0.6 mg/kg body weight. The high dose should be continued until the patient has fully recovered, it may then be stopped immediately, there is no need to 'tail off' the treatment.

An example of systemic steroids is prednisolone. Prednesol is particularly useful for children as it is soluble.

Inhaled steroids

These are now being used extensively in the management of asthma and are extremely successful if taken on a regular prophylactic basis. The doses are minute (200 µg twice daily is a typical dose) and since the drug is delivered straight to the linings of the bronchi and bronchioles, the risks of serious side effects are removed. Inhaled steroids take about 3 – 7 days before they are fully effective and they must be taken on a regular basis. They are of *no* value during an acute attack of asthma. About 5% of people using inhaled steroids develop oropharyngeal thrush and occasionally hoarseness of the voice is noticed.

Examples are beclomethasone (Becotide) and budesonide (Pulmicort). High-dose (250 µg) versions of beclomethasone (Becloforte) are available for more severe asthmatics.

Sodium cromoglycate

It is not fully understood how sodium cromoglycate (Intal) works, although we know that it blocks bronchoconstrictor responses to challenge by exercise and antigen. It is used as a prophylactic agent after an inhaled β_2-stimulant has failed to control the symptoms and it must be used regularly four times a day. It is of particular value to the young atopic asthmatic, and may also be used to prevent exercise-induced asthma in which case a dose may be inhaled half an hour before exercise. Intal is a very safe preparation and the only side-effects appear to be the taste and the tendency to cough after inhaling the dry powder. A high-dose Intal preparation is now available for twice daily administration.

Nedocromil

Nedocromil (Tilade) is a new drug intended for prophylaxis rather than symptomatic relief. It appears to inhibit a variety of mediators which cause inflammation and bronchospasm. It is available in a metered dose inhaler to be used 2 – 4 times a day. It is not recommended for children under 12 years.

Ketotifen

Ketotifen (Zaditen) which is available in tablet form or syrup, is a type of antihistamine and is an oral alternative to sodium cromoglycate. It has not been widely adopted in the United Kingdom as its response is often disappointing. The side-effects can include drowsiness.

Drug combinations

Some of the inhaled drugs are available in fixed combinations which may be useful in some situations. However, the fixed dosage means that prescribing lacks the flexibility which is so often necessary for successful management. Ventide is a combination of typical doses of salbutamol and beclomethasone (β_2-stimulant and inhaled corticosteroid) and can be convenient if patients do not need extra salbutamol. Duovent is a mixture of ipratropium and fenoterol (anticholinergic and β_2-stimulant) and can be helpful to patients who require both. This combination is particularly recommended for patients over 40.

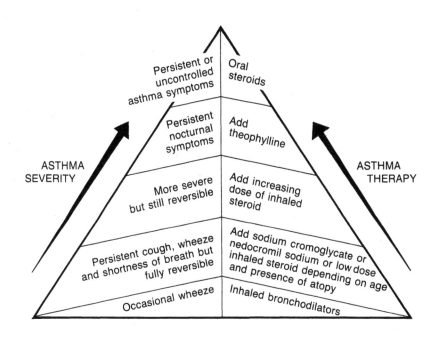

Fig. 5.5 Summary of Asthma Management according to severity.

Delivery systems

There is no doubt that many asthmatics would prefer to take their asthma treatment orally. Swallowing a tablet is less noticeable than using an inhaling device and some people are embarrassed about using a device in public. It is important to explain why asthma treatment is best given by inhalation.

1   Inhaled therapy is transported directly to the bronchi and therefore works much faster than the oral route.
2   The dosage required is considerably smaller, and therefore safer.
3   There are few, if any, side effects.

Over the years many devices have been developed and all the drugs, apart from theophylline, may be given by inhalation. There are times, however, particularly in acute situations, when it is necessary to give corticosteroids orally or by injection. For a minority of patients, oral preparations have to be prescribed because they are incapable of using a device.

Before offering an adequate asthma service, the nurse should obtain working examples of all the different devices for demonstration to the patient. She should also have practised sufficiently with them to be convincing and confident in explanation.

Metered dose inhalers

Metered dose inhalers (Figure 5.6) have been in use for some years and are a very convenient method of delivering the treatment, as long as the patient can simultaneously co-ordinate inspiration with depressing the canister. It is worth noting that 20% of doctors cannot do this!

All treatments for asthma, apart from systemic steroids and theophylline, may be prescribed by metered dose inhalers.

Only one inhalation should be taken at a time and it is usual to wait about half a minute before repeating the exercise.

Aerolin Autohaler

Recently the Aerolin Autohaler (Figure 5.7) has been introduced. No co-ordination is required for this device. The correct dose is automatically fired.

Spacer devices

Extension tubes can be fitted onto metered dose inhalers and these will help overcome the problems of co-ordination. The spacer device (e.g. Nebuhaler, Volumatic) has proved invaluable for giving treatment to the very young, the elderly and the poorly co-ordinated. It has also been found to be useful in reducing the incidence of oral thrush, which may occur with the inhalation of steroids. The spacer will retain most of the larger particles of the drug which would otherwise collect in the patient's mouth.

1. Remove the cap and shake the inhaler.

2. Breathe out gently.

3. Put the mouthpiece in the mouth and at the start of inspiration, which should be slow and deep, press the canister down and continue to inhale deeply.

4. Hold the breath for about 10 seconds.

5. Wait about 30 seconds before taking another inhalation.

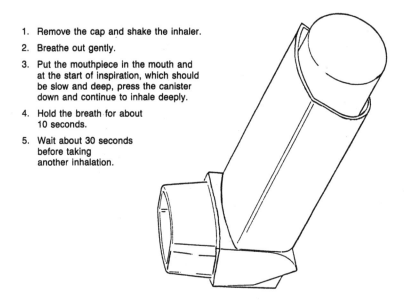

Fig. 5.6   How to use the metered dose inhaler.

1. Remove protective mouthpiece and shake the inhaler.

2. Hold the inhaler upright and push the grey lever right up.

3. Breathe out gently. Keep the inhaler upright and put the mouthpiece in the mouth and close lips round it. (The air holes must not be blocked by the hand.)

4. Breathe in steadily through the mouth. DON'T stop breathing when the inhaler 'clicks' and continue taking a really deep breath.

5. Hold the breath for about 10 seconds.

6. Wait at least 60 seconds before taking another inhalation.

    N.B. The lever must be pushed up ('on') before each dose, and pushed down again ('off') afterwards, otherwise it will not operate.

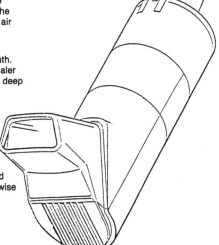

Fig. 5.7   How to use the Autohaler.

The spacer is a plastic, pear-shaped chamber with an inlet for the aerosol at one end and an inspiration valve at the other (Figure 5.8). Once released, the drug is retained in the chamber until the patient breathes in through the mouthpiece when the valve opens and the drug is inspired. On expiration the valve closes and none of the drug can escape.

Fig. 5.8 Volumatic. Instructions for patients who can use the device without help.

1. Remove the cap, shake the inhaler and insert into the device.

2. Place the mouthpiece in the mouth.

3. Press the canister once to release a dose of the drug.

4. Take a deep, slow breath in.

5. Hold the breath for about 10 seconds, then breathe out through the mouthpiece

6. Breathe in again but do not press the canister.

7. Remove the device from the mouth.

8. Wait for 30 seconds before a second dose is taken.

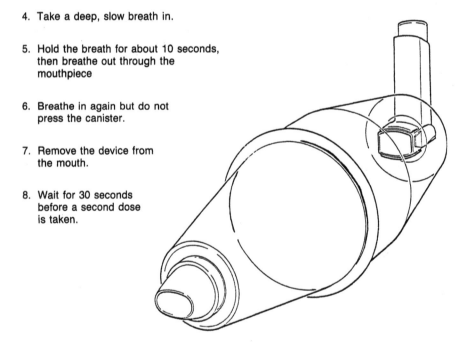

The disadvantage of the spacer device is that it is too bulky to carry around easily and so it is most useful for twice daily prophylactic treatment for which it may be left at home. The Nebuhaler has been designed to be used with terbutaline (Bricanyl) and budesonide (Pulmicort and Pulmicort Paediatric) refill canisters. However it can be used with most other aerosols e.g. sodium cromoglycate (Intal). The Volumatic device should be used with salbutamol (Ventolin) and beclomethasone (Becotide and Becloforte).

These devices are extremely easy to use and mothers with young children (from aged 2 upwards) once instructed in their use usually manage very well (Figure 5.9).

Fig. 5.9 Nebuhaler. Instructions for young children.

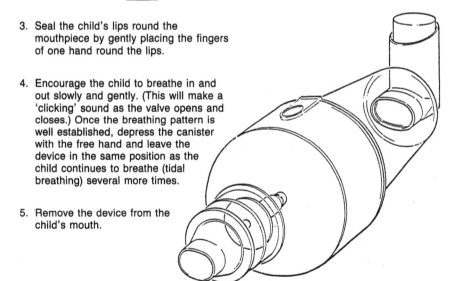

1. Remove the cap, shake the inhaler and insert into the device.

2. Place the mouthpiece in the child's mouth, (if using the Nebuhaler be careful the child's lips are behind the ring).

3. Seal the child's lips round the mouthpiece by gently placing the fingers of one hand round the lips.

4. Encourage the child to breathe in and out slowly and gently. (This will make a 'clicking' sound as the valve opens and closes.) Once the breathing pattern is well established, depress the canister with the free hand and leave the device in the same position as the child continues to breathe (tidal breathing) several more times.

5. Remove the device from the child's mouth.

Remember that either of these methods may be used with both the Volumatic and Nebuhaler devices.

Recently it has been found that very small babies can benefit from using the Nebuhaler device by fixing a small anaesthetic mask on to the inspirational end of the device. When used in this way the Nebuhaler should be pointed downwards after the canister has been depressed so that it is not necessary to activate the valve.

Method of use for severe attacks

Sometimes it may be appropriate to give a larger dose of bronchodilator treatment through the spacer device. For example, instead of using a nebulized bronchodilator for an acute attack, a similar result can often be achieved by assembling the device and inserting a metered dose inhaler. The canister is pressed about 15 times (three puffs at a time) and the patient inhales through the device as in Figure 5.9.

Dry powder devices

There are now a variety of dry powder devices available (Table 5.2, Figure 5.10). All these devices are easy to use and do not require co-ordination. The Triflo is a particularly useful small piece of apparatus which may be used to teach children how to inhale or suck.

Table 5.2 Details of the four main dry powder devices available.

Spinhaler	Sodium cromoglycate (Intal)	Capsules
Rotahaler	Salbutamol (Ventolin) Beclomethasone (Becotide)	Capsules
Diskhaler	Salbutamol (Ventolin) Beclomethasone (Becotide)	Circular foil disks with eight blisters round edge
Turbohaler	Terbutaline (Bricanyl)	Metered dose powder inhaler

1. Hold Spinhaler upright and unscrew
   the body.

2. Put coloured end of the spincap into cup of
   propeller.

3. Screw the two parts together and move
   grey sleeve up and down at least twice,
   this will pierce capsule.

4. Breathe out gently, tilt the head back,
   put Spinhaler into the mouth and
   breathe in quickly and deeply.

5. Remove Spinhaler from the
   mouth and hold breath for
   about 10 seconds.

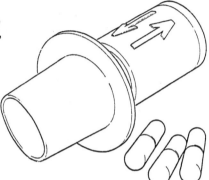

Fig. 5.10 Spinhaler.

1. Hold Rotahaler vertically and put
   capsule coloured end uppermost into
   'square' hole. Make sure top of Rotacap
   is level with top of hole. (If there is a
   Rotacap already in the device this will be
   pushed into shell.)

2. Hold Rotahaler horizontally, twist
   barrel sharply forwards and backwards.
   This splits capsule into two.

3. Breathe out gently. Keep Rotahaler
   level and put mouthpiece between lips
   and teeth and breathe in the powder
   quickly and deeply.

4. Remove Rotahaler from the
   mouth and hold breath for
   about 10 seconds.

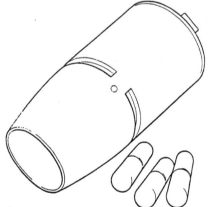

Fig. 5.10(a) Rotahaler.

1. Remove mouthpiece cover. Then remove the white tray by pulling it out gently and then squeezing the white ridges either side until it slides out.

2. Put foil disk – number uppermost – on the wheel and slide tray back.

3. Slide tray in and out by holding the corners of the tray – this will rotate the disk. A number will appear in the small window. Rotate until number 8 appears. As the disk contains 8 doses this is a convenient way of knowing how many doses remain.

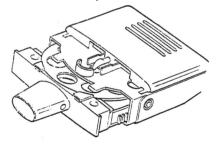

4. Keeping the Diskhaler level, lift the rear of the lid and pull it up as far as it will go. This will pierce the top and bottom of the blister. Close the lid.

5. Hold the Diskhaler level, breathe out gently and put the mouthpiece in the mouth. (Do not cover the small air holes on either side of the mouthpiece.) Breathe in through the mouth as quickly and deeply as possible.

6. Remove the Diskhaler from the mouth and hold the breath for about 10 seconds.

Fig. 5.10(b)   Diskhaler.

1. Unscrew and lift off white cover. Hold Turbohaler upright and twist blue grip forwards and backwards as far as it will go.

2. Breathe out gently, put mouthpiece between the lips and breathe in as deeply as possible.

3. Remove Turbohaler from the mouth and hold breath for about 10 seconds.

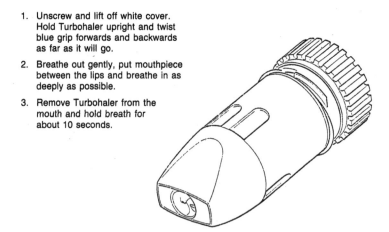

Fig. 5.10(c)   Turbohaler.

Remember that because there are no additives, and there is often no taste, some patients may *feel* that they are not receiving the full dose.

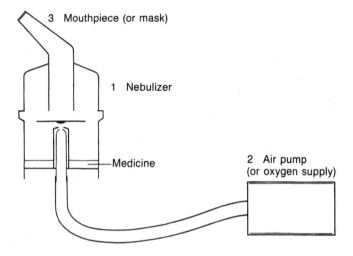

Fig. 5.11 The nebulizer.

Nebulized therapy

One of the drawbacks of most of the inhaler devices is that it is necessary to be able to inhale deeply. Sometimes the patient has a very low inspirational volume, for example in acute asthma, and some other method of giving the treatment is required. The device that creates least resistance to breathing is the nebulizer. This is a device which creates a mist out of a liquid by blowing air or oxygen through it (Figure 5.11). The nebulizer unit consists of:

1 A small container into which a liquid solution of the drug is put and through which air or oxygen can be blown to make the mist.
2 A source of compressed gas, e.g. oxygen or a small electric pump.
3 A mouthpiece or mask which can be attached to the outlet from the nebuilizer so the mist can be inhaled.

Nebulizers can deliver treatment whilst the patient is breathing quietly as no co-operation is required. The dosages of most treatments given via the nebulizer are much higher than those given by other devices, e.g. 2.5 mg of salbutamol may be given as a single nebulized dose which is the equivalent of 25 puffs from a metered dose inhaler. Nebulizers can be used to administer salbutamol (Ventolin), terbutaline (Bricanyl), ipratropium bromide (Atrovent), sodium cromoglycate (Intal), beclomethasone (Becotide) and budesonide (Pulmicort).

Nebulizers are mainly used for:

1 The emergency treatment of acute asthma. A PEFR measurement should be recorded before and after the treatment so that any objective improvement may be measured.
2 Regular treatment of chronic asthma with bronchodilator therapy.
3 Giving preventive treatment to small children.
4 Demonstrating whether significant reversibility of airway resistance is possible in patients with chronic obstructive airways disease (such as chronic bronchitis).

It must be remembered that whilst nebulizers have saved many lives, they can be potentially dangerous when used unsupervised. Some patients who have their own nebulizers place too much faith in them and fail to send for the doctor until it is too late. It is very important if patients need to use the nebulizer twice in 24 hours that they are assessed by a doctor. A course of steroids will usually be required, and the need for admission considered.

Patient education

To educate the asthmatic and his or her family successfully, teaching guidelines have to be agreed. They should be simple and certain criteria followed. A little verbal information which can be absorbed easily by a patient, backed up by written instructions and leaflets is far more effective than a lengthy monologue delivered by the educator. It is important that time is allowed to listen to the patient and to answer any queries. Perhaps the most important messages to get through to patients and their families are:

1 If prophylactic treatment has been prescribed it *must* be taken.
2 Until sufficient knowledge has been acquired about their own condition it is enough to follow instructions.
3 Patients must know they have easy access to advice.

Knowing what to do and when, is of considerably more practical value to the asthmatic than understanding the pathophysiology of the disease.

The nurse is in a good position to teach patients and parents about asthma as she is seen by the public as both approachable and knowledgeable and yet not as important or as busy as the doctor. Asthma patients frequently underestimate and minimize their symptoms and problems, and are unwilling to disturb the doctor with what they consider to be trivialities. Many patients are happier to contact the nurse with what they see as minor problems before they become too major.

How can asthma care be improved?

In order to improve asthma care a special anticipatory and organizational approach needs to be adopted, so that preventive care can be effectively integrated with therapeutic care. It is necessary to know:

1 Who suffers from the condition.
2 How to develop a logical systematic and prophylactic approach to treatment.
3 How to organize follow-up.

It is also important to assess the response to treatment constantly, and to check on compliance. Apart from educating the patient we need to provide on-going support to maintain the patient's trust and enthusiasm.

Extension of the nurse's role

Whilst improving the care of asthma and other chronic disorders certainly benefits the patient, it will also increase the workload of the practice (Figure 5.12). This can be met by extending the role of the practice nurse. If the

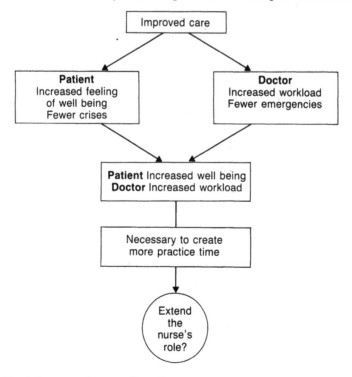

Fig. 5.12 Asthma care in general practice.

nurse is to play a major role in asthma care and patient education, it is important she has the relevant skills. As well as being highly motivated, she needs to have good clinical and organizational abilities and to have a particular interest in the preventative aspects of the condition. Both empathy and skilful communication are vital in dealing successfully with both patients and parents. To what extent each individual nurse's role expands (as detailed below) will depend on many factors, but will largely be dependent upon the nurse's ability and what is acceptable to the doctor, as well as available time and resources.

Minimum involvement

1 Record PEFR.
2 Demonstrate and check inhaler technique.
3 Set up asthma register.

Patient always sees general practitioner, there is no special clinic.

Medium involvement

1 Record PEFR.
2 Demonstrate and check inhaler technique.
3 Set up asthma register.
4 Carry out *tests* (reversibility, exercise).
5 Teach PEFR home-monitoring with diary cards.
6 Improve asthma education.
7 Give explanatory literature.

Could lead to doctor and nurse asthma clinic review.

Maximum involvement

1 Record PEFR.
2 Demonstrate and check inhaler technique.
3 Set up asthma register.
4 Carry out test (reversibility, exercise).
5 Teach PEFR home-monitoring with diary cards.
6 Improve asthma education.
7 Give explanatory literature.
8 Carry out assessment and regular follow-up.
9 Formulate projected structured treatment plan.
10 Write prescriptions (signed by doctor after discussion).
11 Give advice by telephone.
12 See patient in an emergency.

Nurse-run asthma clinic review with doctor advice as required.

For both minimum and medium nurse involvement the doctor's co-operation and the nurse's capability are likely to be complementary since the nurse is not infringing on the doctor's territory. If it is agreed that the nurse's role should extend to maximal level and the nurse should be responsible for running an asthma clinic, then not only does she require support and advice from the doctor, but there needs to be considerable mutual confidence and trust between the members of the two professions. Good teamwork is essential for this care to work effectively. The nurse's role will develop with experience and increased confidence. However, it is not recommended that a nurse should attempt maximal involvement without first attending an in-depth, training programme in asthma care.

Appendix: Useful addresses

The Asthma Society Training Centre

22 Scholars Lane
Stratford-upon-Avon
Warwickshire
CV37 6HE

Since April 1987, the Asthma Society Training Centre in Stratford-upon-Avon has been training practice nurses in the management of asthma in general practice. Nurses attend a 3-day in-depth course and one of their general practitioners attends on the final day. The objective of the course is to improve the standard of care of asthmatics within the community by equipping doctors and nurses with the logical, systematic approach necessary for effective care.

The course programme covers all the aspects of asthma mangement. These include:

- asthma—the disease and diagnosis;
- the treatment and management of asthma;
- practical procedures;
- overall structured policies and guidelines;
- practice organization, including audit;
- consultations with asthmatic patients;
- use of video recorder in consultation analysis;
- 'adept' computer diagnostic training aid.

Approximately 40 courses are held yearly, with ten nurses attending each course. Many nurses have demonstrated, on return to their practices, an excellent understanding of asthma and the care of asthmatic patients. Undoubtedly, the nurses most likely to continue developing and extending their role in this field have been those where the doctor also attended the course.

Both the course director (Greta Barnes) and the medical tutor (Dr Robert Pearson) also work at Bridge House Medical Centre, Stratford-upon-Avon and the training programme is based upon the Asthma Care Programme developed in the practice.

National Asthma Campaign *(formerly Asthma Society and Friends of the Asthma Research Council)*

300 Upper Street
London
N1 2XX

A free professional pack of asthma literature is available; as are peak flow meters (priced £8.00 to include post and packing).

Acknowledgements

My thanks to Bob Pearson for permission to reproduce two of his diagrams and also for his help and unfailing patience and instruction over the past 6 years.

Further reading

Clark, T. J. J. & Godfrey, S. (eds) (1983) *Asthma*, 2nd edn. Chapman & Hall, London.
Clark, T. J. J. & Rees, J. (1985) *Practical Management of Asthma*. Martin Dunitz, London.
Pearson, R. (1990) *Asthma Care in General Practice*. Radcliffe Medical Press, Oxford.
Rees, J. & Price, J. (1989) *ABC of Asthma*. BMJ Publications, London.

6 Care of Patients with Hypertension

HYPERTENSION is a treatable chronic disease. Its manifestations include cerebrovascular haemorrhage or infarction, renal failure, plus coronary heart and peripheral arterial diseases. These secondary consequences, which are also associated with high blood lipids and smoking, are responsible for more premature deaths than any other cause, including cancer and infection combined.

Severe hypertension, with diastolics over 130 mmHg, is found in 0.5% of the population aged between 35 and 65 years. Moderate hypertension, with diastolic pressures between 110 and 129 mmHg, is found in 4 – 5% of adults. Milder grades of hypertension, with diastolic pressures of between 90 and 109 mmHg, are found in about 20% of the middle-aged population. A casual blood pressure of over 160/95 is found in 50% of over seventies.

These figures, however, are all based on population screening surveys using a single casual blood pressure recording. Many of these high readings will fall on rechecking (Beevers 1982), probably because of reduced fear in the patient or better technique by the observer. Indeed a large American survey only identified 6% of the population with diastolic pressures persistently above 90 mmHg (Hypertension Detection and Follow-up Program Co-operative Group 1979). This illustrates the absolute need for repeated blood pressure estimations, the adequate training of observers and the proper maintenance of accurate recording equipment.

Definition

Probably the most precise definition of hypertension is the level of blood pressure above which investigation and treatment is of proven value to the patient (Grimley Evans & Rose 1971). This encompasses the dilemma over what actually constitutes an abnormal blood pressure (BP) level and the need to balance the individual's risk of developing complications against the side effects of investigation or treatment. Although these considerations should not be ignored, perhaps a more pragmatic definition of hypertension is needed. This is best served by the World Health Organization (WHO) criteria (1978) listed in Table 6.1. There are additional points to consider with these criteria:

- diastolic readings are phase V (disappearance of sounds);
- abnormal readings should occur on repeated examination (at least three examinations);

- the age of the patient should be considered (these figures only refer to under seventies);
- existence of vascular complications of hypertension would lower the threshold for treatment.

Table 6.1 WHO criteria for hypertension.

	Systolic BP	Diastolic BP
Normal	<140	<90
Borderline	140 – 159 *and/or*	90 – 94
Definite	160 + *and/or*	95 +
Mild hypertension	160 – 179 *and/or*	95 – 104

Physiology of blood pressure

It is important to have a basic understanding of the physiology of blood pressure in order to understand how it varies, how the drugs used in treatment work, and also to be able to explain blood pressure simply and clearly to patients. There are several physiological components that affect the blood pressure.

1 *The heart.* With each beat it pumps blood from the left ventricle into the aorta. This raises the BP to peak or systolic pressure. Blood pressure increases with the rate, force and volume of each beat.
2 *The aorta and other large arteries* dilate to receive each pulse of blood. If the walls of these vessels are more rigid the systolic pressure will be higher.
3 *The peripheral arteries* allow the blood to run out of the aorta into the arterioles and capillaries. These vessels contain smooth muscle which can contract to narrow the blood vessels and increase the blood pressure.
4 *The kidney* produces a hormone (renin) which in turn converts angiotensin to an active hormone. This causes constriction of the blood vessels and affects the retention of salt and fluid by the kidney, increasing the total blood volume.

The level of BP is controlled by the sympathetic nervous system which has two groups of effects, classified as alpha and beta. Stimulation of beta-receptors increases the heart rate and the strength of the heart's contraction. Stimulation of the alpha-receptors causes constriction of the blood vessels. The level of sympathetic activity required to maintain the BP is controlled by baroreceptors. These are specialized nerve endings in the carotid arteries sensitive to the pressure in the vessel.

Each person's blood pressure varies around the base line level. It goes up with exertion and anxiety, and is reduced by rest. Blood pressure is higher when standing than sitting or lying down. The factors that influence a resting blood pressure include the following.

1   *Heredity.* This is the largest single factor that explains the difference in blood pressures between individuals. This might explain 50% of BP variation.

2   *Age.* The average blood pressure of the population increases with age. Systolic BP increases more because of the loss of elasticity of the arteries. If your blood pressure is higher when you are younger, it will increase more with age and people with lower blood pressures may have very little increase at all (this means that patients with marginally raised blood pressures should be followed up more frequently).

3   *Weight.* There is strong relationship between increased weight and BP. This can be reversed on losing weight.

4   *Alcohol intake.* Many studies have demonstrated a direct relationship between alcohol consumption and hypertension. There is also a close correlation between high alcohol intake and stroke.

5   *Salt.* Populations which have a high salt diet have a higher average BP, but it is more difficult to demonstrate that this is true for individuals.

6   *Drug-induced.* Nearly all women taking the combined contraceptive pill have a very small rise in BP. A significant rise may occur in up to 5% of patients. Hormone replacement therapy (HRT) also may raise blood pressure. Oral corticosteroids produce hypertension in high doses, but do not appear to cause problems in chronic low dosage. Non-steroidal anti-inflammatories like indomethacin may cause hypertension secondary to fluid retention.

7   *Secondary hypertension.* There are a small number of people (under 5%) whose BP is raised because of other disease. These include renal disease (such as polycystic kidneys or renal artery stenosis), coarctation of the aorta, and endocrine diseases like Cushing's disease (due to excess cortisol), primary hyperaldosteronism (excess aldosterone) or phaeochromocytoma (excess adrenaline or noradrenaline). Secondary hypertension is more likely to be the cause in younger patients with high BP.

There is very little convincing data that the following are implicated in hypertension: potassium levels, stress, cigarette smoking, coffee, calcium or trace metals.

Consequences of raised blood pressure

A raised blood pressure affects the body in a number of ways.

The heart

The incidence of angina and myocardial infarction (MI) are both doubled. Compared to normotensives, about 1% of hypertensives suffer an MI each year.

The wall of the left ventricle may also become thickened. This left ventricular hypertrophy is related to the level of blood pressure. It occurs in 5% of patients with moderate hypertension (diastolic BP 110 – 120 mmHg) and has a poor prognosis (Kannel 1965). Compared to a similarly severe hypertensive with no hypertrophy the risk of heart attack is increased fourfold, stroke 12-fold and claudication threefold.

The arteries

High blood pressure contributes to the development of atheroma, which in turn can lead to heart attacks, strokes and peripheral artery disease.

The arterioles may become narrowed due to vasoconstriction. This may damage renal and cerebral function; produce aneurysms which may burst and cause a haemorrhagic stroke; or rarely develop acute inflammation or fibrinoid necrosis, causing malignant or accelerated hypertension. This is a rapidly fatal condition if untreated.

The brain

Around 50% of patients with subarachnoid haemorrhage have hypertension. This presents as acute severe headache with meningism and altered consciousness. About half of the patients will die with their first haemorrhage. Hypertension also contributes to the incidence of cerebral aneurysms which occur in 70% of subarachnoids.

Cerebral haemorrhage is a common complication in severe hypertension. This is the commonest cause of stroke amongst blacks. Strokes in whites are more likely to be due to cerebral infarcts. These infarcts occur with less severe hypertension, due to atheroma of the intracranial vessels.

The overall risk of stroke is around half that of suffering an MI with an incidence of 2% when diastolic BP is above 110 mmHg and 0.5% per year when diastolic BP is around 100 mmHg.

The kidney

Untreated hypertension leads to progressive renal damage, due to arteriosclerosis, and eventually renal failure. Death from renal failure is five times that in normotensives. Seventy percent of patients on renal dialysis have hypertension. Mild haematuria and proteinuria is common and should be monitored by blood urea and creatinine levels.

Significance of hypertension

Hypertension is the commonest and single most powerful predictor of premature death from arterial disease, and the following points need to be considered.

1 *Incidence.* This is greatest in patients aged 35 – 65 years. There is a 5% incidence amongst people with diastolic blood pressures greater than 110 mmHg, and 20% incidence for diastolic blood pressures of 90 – 109 mmHg.
2 *Absolute risk.* This increases with age. The 2-year death rates are:
   - 60%—severe hypertension (diastolic BP >130 mmHg);
   - 20%—moderate hypertension (diastolic BP 100 – 129 mmHg);
   - 1 – 3%—mild hypertension (diastolic BP 95 – 110 mmHg).
3 *Multiple risk factors.* The risk of hypertension is greatly increased in patients who smoke or have raised lipids. Table 6.2 illustrates the varying annual death rates in patients with multiple risk factors. These are for men aged between 35 and 45 years; they are much higher in older patients.
4 *High risk groups.* If we wish to identify which patients are at particular risk of having a heart attack, and take high blood pressure alone we can only identify one-third of potential patients. However, if we score all the risk factors together then over half of the coronary heart disease deaths will occur in the top 20% of those at risk.

Moderate or severe hypertension is a major risk factor in its own right and requires treatment. The significance of mild hypertension depends on the presence or absence of other risk factors.

Table 6.2 Annual death rates in patients with multiple risk factors for hypertension.

Risk factor	Annual death rate/thousand
Hypertension with diastolic BP >90 mmHg	4
Hypertension with cholesterol >6.2 mmol/l	10
Hypertension with smoking	11
Hypertension with smoking and high lipids	17

Taking the blood pressure

Because decisions about treatment are made on small differences in blood pressure it is important that it is taken consistently and accurately. The important points to remember are:

- the patient should be sitting comfortably with their arm supported;
- the cuff should be applied at the level of the heart and there should not be any tight clothing constricting the arm above it;
- if a cuff is used that is too small for the arm, the recorded BP will be too high. The standard cuff should be marked with an upper limit circumference (13 inches, 275 mm) and if this is exceeded a larger cuff should be used;
- the cuff must be inflated above the systolic BP and this should be checked by feeling the pulse;
- blood pressure should be measured to the nearest 2 mmHg;
- the systolic BP is when the blood pressure sounds are first heard, and diastolic pressure should be recorded at phase V when the sounds disappear.

Common sources of error when taking blood pressure are:

1 A machine which is poorly maintained. The column should be vertical, clean and the mercury should rest at 0 mmHg when deflated.
2 The observer may

- deflate the column too quickly;
- read the blood pressure to the nearest 5 or 10 mmHg;
- be biased to record a preconceived result.

3 The patient may be unduly anxious, particularly with a new observer.

Assessing the patient

There are several questions which need to be asked when assessing a patient with possible hypertension.

1 *Is the blood pressure consistently raised?* Decisions to initiate treatment should be taken on the mean of three readings taken on separate occasions at 2 – 4-weekly intervals.
2 *Is there any possible cause for the elevation?* Exclude drug precipitants.
3 *Is there any end organ damage?* Check for a history of angina, claudication or shortness of breath. Examine the cardiovascular system and fundi. Investigate the urine and perform an ECG.

4 *Are any other risk factors present?* Question about alcohol intake, smoking, diet and physical activity. Exclude diabetes or hypercholesterolaemia.

5 *Are there any factors to influence the choice of treatment?* Consider a history of angina, asthma, gout or depression. Consider checking the blood glucose and uric acid.

Initial investigations should therefore include a urine test, full blood count, profile (and possibly random cholesterol) and an ECG. Further investigations are only justified in young patients or those who fail to respond to treatment. Some patients should be referred for specialist review:

- patients under 45 years;
- severe hypertensives with diastolic BP above 125 mmHg;
- hypertension not controlled by two drugs in combination;
- signs of primary cause or of complications.

Further investigations on such patients may include intravenous urography, 24-hour urine tests for catecholamines or blood hormone levels.

Who should be treated?

It has been already stated that there is no 'disease' of hypertension which some patients have and others do not. The decision to start treatment is based on a balance of its costs, risks and side effects on the one hand and the benefits, which have been established in clinical trials, on the other.

The conclusions from these trials are as follows.

1 Patients whose diastolic BP is above 105 mmHg on three occasions should be encouraged to take treatment.

2 Patients whose blood pressures are 90 – 105 mmHg should be observed for 3 – 4 months. If the diastolic pressure remains over 100 mmHg they should be offered treatment.

3 Presence of end organ damage or other risk factors such as hyperlipidaemia, diabetes, a strong family history of heart disease or smokers (who cannot be persuaded to stop) should encourage treatment earlier and at lower levels.

4 More elderly patients have raised blood pressures and they are more prone to experience side effects from treatment. Their risk of stroke, however, is much higher and the potential benefits to the individual patient of treatment is correspondingly greater. There is, therefore, no justification for withholding antihypertensive drugs from the elderly (at least those under 80) on the grounds of age alone.

The evidence from all the trials is that if good control is achieved (diastolic BP below 90 mmHg) the patient's risk of stroke is reduced to normal. There is less reduction in the risk of heart disease, which may depend on prolonged treatment and more attention to other risk factors.

Management

The aims of management are to reduce the patient's blood pressure and their overall risk of heart disease and stroke, while maintaining or improving their quality of life. The important ingredients are as follows.

1 *Stopping smoking.* Probably the single most important thing that can be done for a patient with high blood pressure.
2 *Dietary advice.* The principle aim is to reduce weight to normal levels and hence lower the blood pressure. Specific advice should be offered on dietary modification such as: reduce salt intake (stop adding salt to food); avoid processed foods like bacon, sausages or snacks like peanuts or crisps; increase roughage with fruit, vegetables and cereals; and reduce fat intake (substitute polyunsaturates for saturated fats). These dietary changes will not only improve blood pressure but will reduce additional risk factors.
3 *Reduce alcohol intake.* This will lower the blood pressure, particularly if the intake was previously excessive (greater than 12 units/week in women or 25 units/week in men).
4 *Regular exercise.* This may have particular effect on the coronary arteries but also increases the patient's well-being and counteracts any belief that they now have an illness. Exercise should be dynamic (swimming, running, cycling) not isometric (weights in gym).

Antihypertensive drugs

It will be helpful to refer back to the section on the physiology of blood pressure to understand the mechanism of the action of drugs. There are four main groups of hypertensive drugs: thiazide diuretics and beta-blockers, which are well established and usually regarded as first-line drugs, plus calcium antagonists and ACE inhibitors, which have been introduced more recently. The choice of drug should depend on the individual patient. Factors to consider include:

- effectiveness in controlling hypertension;
- possible contraindications;
- cost;
- type or frequency of side effects.

Thiazide diurectics

1 *Examples*. Bendrofluazide 2.5 mg, hydroclorthiazide 12.5 – 25 mg daily.
2 *Mode of action*. Act on the kidney tubules to block sodium reabsorption. This produces a slight loss of total body water and a commensurate reduction in plasma volume, reducing the blood pressure. The effect is counteracted by a reflex rise in renin and angiotensin (renal enzymes) and this prevents further falls of blood pressure. For this reason, there is no point in increasing the dose of the diuretic if full control is not achieved by the stated dosages.
3 *Important side effects*. Reduces serum potassium (only add potassium supplements if potassium falls below 3.5 mmol/l), raises serum uric acid (possibly precipitating gout), raises blood sugar (precipitating diabetes), and can cause impotence.
4 *Particular indications*. Heart failure, elderly patients.
5 *Contraindications*. Diabetes, renal failure, gout, impotence.

Beta-blockers

1 *Examples*. Propranolol 160 mg or atenolol 50 – 100 mg daily.
2 *Mode of action*. Block the adrenergic β-receptors thereby preventing their stimulation by catecholamines (adrenaline and noradrenaline). β_1-receptor blockade reduces the heart rate and contractility, thereby reducing cardiac output. β_2-blockade produces vasodilatation dropping blood pressure, but also can cause bronchoconstriction in susceptible individuals. Further BP reduction may occur to the inhibition of renin and angiotensin release. Cardioselective β-blockers (atenolol, metoprolol) have most of their effect on type 1 β-receptors. Non-selective blockers (propranolol, oxprenolol) have an equal effect on type 1 and 2 receptors.
3 *Side effects*. Bronchospasm, due to β_2-receptor blockade; heart failure or fatiguability, due to reduction in cardiac contractility; cold extremities, due to reduced cardiac output and reflex peripheral vasoconstriction; central nervous system effects (lethargy, nightmares and poor sleep), due to blockers which are lipid-soluble and cross the blood – brain barrier (propranolol, oxprenolol).
4 *Particular indications*. Angina.
5 *Contraindications*. Asthma, heart failure, peripheral vascular disease, insulin-dependent diabetes, depression.

Calcium antagonists

1 *Examples*. Nifedipine 10 – 20 mg b.d. verapamil 80 – 160 mg b.d.
2 *Mode of action*. Reduce the amount of free calcium in the cell thereby relaxing arteriolar smooth muscle and producing vasodilatation.

3 *Side effects.* Vary according to the particular calcium antagonist. Verapamil may produce constipation and occasionally facial flushing. Nifedipine commonly causes facial flushing and occasionally headaches or lower limb oedema (due to local tissue inflammation not water retention).

4 *Particular indications.* Peripheral vascular disease, angina, severe hypertension.

5 *Contraindications.* Heart failure.

Angiotensin-converting enzyme (ACE) inhibitors

1 *Examples.* Enalapril 2.5 – 20 mg daily or b.d., captopril 12.5 – 50 mg b.d.

2 *Mode of action.* Block the enzymes in the renin – angiotensin system preventing the formation of angiotensin II, thereby inhibiting vasoconstriction.

3 *Side effects.* Large drop in BP in patients previously taking a loop diuretic (such as frusemide). First dose effect (precipitate drop in BP with first tablet). Drug should be started in a very low dose and diuretics (especially loop) preferably withdrawn. Patients with renal damage may develop leucopenia and proteinuria, occasional skin rashes or persistent cough.

4 *Particular indications.* Heart failure, side effects from other drugs.

5 *Contraindications.* Renal failure, high doses of diuretics (patients should be referred for hospital stabilization).

If a single drug does not decrease blood pressure sufficiently, these drugs may be used in combination. The combinations which are particularly effective are thiazides and β-blockers, thiazides and ACE inhibitors, or β-blockers and nifedipine. There is no benefit from increasing the dose of β-blockers and thiazides used together. However, raising the diuretic dose with ACE drugs will increase the hypotensive effect. Verapamil should not be prescribed alongside a β-blocker.

Other drugs, now rarely used, include methyldopa, clonidine, α-receptor blockers (like prazosin) or vasodilators (like hydralazine or minoxidil).

The practice nurse and hypertension

Of all the chronic diseases managed in primary care, hypertension is perhaps the one where the role of the nurse is best established. It is well recognized that nurses will follow a protocol reliably. This is an important factor in a condition where the measure of control is so easy to ascertain but where abnormal values are then frequently ignored. The practice nurse is ideally placed to monitor and run clinics. Before nurses can help with the management of patients with hypertension they require more training since general nurse education does not deal with blood pressure in enough depth. There are now many more opportunities for nurses to acquire this training. This training should include:

- natural history of hypertension and its complications;
- management options including how the drugs work and what side effects may occur;
- practical aspects, such as how to take the BP reading correctly (what size cuff, positioning of the arm), venepuncture and interpretation of blood results;
- ECG recording;
- patient education;
- the role at primary and secondary prevention;
- how to set about developing and running blood pressure clinics.

Organization of care

To achieve the detection, assessment, management and follow-up of patients with high blood pressure in general practice requires careful organization. The ingredients of this organization are:

1 protocol of the practice policies;
2 records of patient care;
3 register to identify patients with high blood pressure;
4 performance review or audit.

Protocol

This should cover the following areas:

- the method of detecting high BP in existing and new patients;
- technique for taking blood pressure (e.g. phase IV or V diastolic);
- verification of hypertension;
- indications for treatment;
- methods of risk factor reduction;
- choice of drugs and indications for referral;
- resources for patient education;
- frequency of follow-up;
- contribution of the practice nurse in detection, management and follow-up.

Record card

A structured record card or flow sheet (Figure 6.1) should reflect the practice protocol and should assist prompt adherence to this protocol. It presents necessary information each time the patient is seen and enables the quality of care and control to be audited.

Practice register

This could be anything from a simple card index kept in date order, to a file on the practice computer. It should identify two main groups of patients: (1) patients whose blood pressures have been found to be raised and require follow-up; and (2) patients who have been started on treatment. In both cases it should indicate when they were last seen or are due for further follow-up.

Performance review

The purpose of reviewing performance is to establish the degree to which one has met one's aims; to be encouraged by increasing success to make changes when they are seen to be required. A sample of the patient's records selected at random is often sufficient. The questions that might be asked include the following.

1 *For the practice population over 35 years.* What percentage of patients have had their BP taken in the last 5 years? Of those with a recorded BP greater than 90 mmHg, what proportion have been followed-up or treated? What proportion of these patients also have records of weight or smoking habits?
2 *For patients started on treatment.* How many blood pressures were recorded before treatment was started? Is the patient's weight and smoking history recorded? What proportion of treated patients have diastolic blood pressures less than 90 mmHg? What proportion of patients are no longer receiving treatment or follow-up?

Protocol development

A protocol needs to be developed to clarify the aims and objectives within each practice. Ideally, everyone who is to deal with the patient should be involved in contributing to this. It is used as the source of reference for day-to-day guidance. It is important not to allow any difficulties in producing a protocol to hinder further practice development of improved care for its

HYPERTENSION RECORD		RISK FACTORS	Habit	Agreed Goals	PATIENT EDUCATION	Given
Date Of Starting Treatment ..../..../....		Smoking			Nature Of Raised BP	
Pre-Treatment BPS — Date	Blood Pressure	Alcohol			Benefits Of Treatment	
1 ..../..../....	/	Exercise			Regimen & Life Style	
2 ..../..../....	/	Diet			Follow Up & Compliance	
3 ..../..../....	/				Reporting Side Effects	
PAST HISTORY No Yes		ASSESSMENTS Initial : Periodic at .... yearly intervals.				
Angina		Date				
Claudication		ECG				
MI		CVS				
CVA		Fundi				
Other		U & E				
FAMILY HISTORY No Yes		Cholesterol				
Hypertension		Triglycerides				
Diabetes		Urate				
Heart Disease		Blood Sugar				
C V Disease		MSU				
Other						

Fig. 6.1 Hypertension record card.

RISK FACTORS:-				TARGETS:- Height · BP · Weight	MANAGEMENT:-			
DATE	P	WT	RISK FACTORS	BP	70 80 90 100 110 120 130 140 150 160 170 180 190 200	Symptoms: Side Effects: Compliance: R	N	Dr

hypertensives. However, the long-term benefits once a protocol has been decided should not be underestimated. Any protocol will need to consider the following areas.

Policy for case finding

- Which patients at risk should be screened?
- Method of screening?
- Follow-up of defaulters?
- What information is wanted?

The practice will need to decide on the age of the groups to be screened. A statement is needed on how these patients are going to be screened: opportunistically when they attend the surgery for some other reason, or by specific invitation to a Well Person clinic? What ought to be done about defaulters, or patients with borderline levels of blood pressure? A decision about additional patient information should debate the levels of BP considered abnormal, and include smoking and alcohol history, weight and family history.

Technique for taking blood pressure

If both doctors and nurses are taking and recording blood pressures, it is important for these recordings to be consistent by standardizing:

1 the type of sphygmomanometer;
2 the position of the patient;
3 the size of the cuffs;
4 the phase for reading the diastolic pressure.

Verification of high blood pressure

The decision to initiate treatment should be based on the mean of at least three readings, taken over a period of several weeks. Even when there is severe hypertension, these three readings should still be taken but over a shorter period. The only exception is malignant hypertension which is very rare. This has other signs (severe headaches, altered consciousness) and has a diastolic usually in excess of 140 mmHg. It is a medical emergency requiring urgent treatment.

Indications for intervention

Decide what information is necessary to proceed to different levels of treatment, be they drugs, risk factor reduction or observation. For the blood pressure consider what level the team accepts as normal, definitely hypertensive and borderline. Decide what method is used to assess weight (body mass index or Garrow chart) and what to do about those overweight. The place of lipids is increasingly important. Who ought to have cholesterol measured? This might be all hypertensives or could be certain groups with other identified risk factors. What lipid level is considered normal or abnormal, and what advice and follow-up is required?

Risk factors

What are the aims of the team in relation to smoking, weight, diet, alcohol and exercise? Consistent advice is the goal. This will ultimately be achieved by finding out what the patient knows, active listening, negotiation of goals and involvement of the patient in monitoring and follow-up. Knowledge of additional risk factors requires follow-up. Decide when health education should be reinforced or progress monitored.

Drugs and referral to doctor

The protocol should preferably state what drugs are to be used. This will probably be in a tiered structure, depending upon age, sex and smoking history of the patient. It should also clearly indicate what factors dictate the need to see a doctor. These might include increase of symptoms or new symptoms, shortness of breath, claudication, angina, non-compliance, side effects or unsatisfactory blood pressure control.

Outside help and reinforcement

Additional information might be advised, such as health education literature. It is useful to provide lists of local amenities, including slimming clubs or sports facilities. Awareness of healthier products available in local supermarkets is also worth adding.

Follow-up monitoring

The protocol must address the frequency of review; details to be monitored; levels of control considered acceptable; role of further investigations; and the point for starting secondary treatment or referral. Further decisions should be taken on the recall of patients with borderline hypertension or poor compliers with treatment.

The nursing role

Once the aims, objectives and methods (the protocol) have been developed, the nurse will feel more confident in developing her own role. It ought to have been decided what the nursing consultation should include, such as discussing long-term aims with the patient, eliciting their existing knowledge, educating, counselling, supporting and follow-up. In addition, practical areas such as taking the blood pressure, checking for risk factors and taking ECGs also need to be considered. It also ought to have been decided at what points the doctor is involved in the ongoing management of these patients.

The practice will need to decide how the nursing involvement is to be introduced. Are there enough nursing hours and rooms within the practice to allow for a nurse-run clinic? Does the practice require another nurse to allow for this greater involvement? It is vital to provide protected time; that is time set aside to allow the nursing consultation to take on sufficient depth to promote education, counselling, support and follow-up. Not all practices will want or require lengthy clinics, but some time must be allocated specifically for each patient. It is not really possible to fit it in with routine, task-orientated treatment room work.

Hypertensive patients can be grouped as follows:

- known hypertensives taking medication;
- newly diagnosed hypertensives;
- borderline group;
- patients new to the practice list;
- for follow-up if known to be hypertensive;
- for screening, an essential part of BP management.

If these groups are not easily identified by computer or established registers, the practice would need to compile a list. This can be composed from repeat prescriptions for antihypertensives, and by doctors and nurses adding to the list all newly diagnosed and borderline patients. Eventually a register of hypertensives will ensue.

Within the protocol it should have been agreed how often the patients need to be seen. Preferably this will include an initial nursing appointment and then alternative appointments between the doctor and the nurse to allow for continuity of care from both disciplines. Decisions also need to be made as to how the patient is informed of this extra involvement by the nurse. Their doctor could explain at the next routine appointment or the patient could be sent details, again from the patient's own doctor, with an explanation and appointment time. The latter method means that a mini-clinic could be established more quickly. Eventually, as all patients are seen, the need to send letters would end since all newly diagnosed hypertensives would filter straight into the established system.

Having finally got the patient through the system, what next? Patients in the practice may be used to consulting the nurse, or it may be a completely new approach for them. They may not necessarily agree that it is for the best and may prefer all their care to come from their own doctor. Their wishes must be respected. However, if they are less willing to be seen it may be useful to explain the aims of the clinic and the nursing input.

Initially the patient needs to feel welcome and comfortable (see Chapter 3 on communication). The explanation of aims often enables the patient to relax and take in the surroundings for a few moments. This discussion may cover the following aspects:

- the need to achieve a target blood pressure;
- highlighting of risk factors;
- offer of support with risk factor reduction;
- the place of regular routine investigations;
- organization of regular follow-up.

To achieve these aims, the provision of care can be considered in four stages. This approach is not unique to caring for the hypertensive patients, since it is the basis for all good consultations.

1 Explore the patient's ideas.
2 React to those ideas.
3 Negotiate goals.
4 Follow-up and support.

Such consultations may be complex and a lot of information about the patient will need to be made available. To clarify this process it is helpful to have a flow chart which incorporates relevant information. This will highlight specific risk factors and provides a record of advice given and goals set. This ensures continuity of care, and clearly identifies those aspects yet to be covered. In establishing the flow chart, information will be gleaned from the patient's medical records as well as acquiring additional information directly.

Having covered the overall aims listed above and using an appropriate means of recording the information, consideration of the condition and the identification of any risk factors can be discussed with the patients.

Initial consultation

This should focus upon the patient's understanding of their condition before any modification of their behaviour is contemplated. They need to appreciate the anatomy and physiology of the circulatory system to appreciate how the risk factors affect their condition before they can choose to make changes to their lifestyle. These consultations should address the following areas:

- the nature of blood pressure;
- benefits of treatment;
- regimen and lifestyle;
- follow-up and compliance;
- reporting side effects.

Collect as much information as you can using open-ended questions, listening attentively and responding as appropriate. Tell me what you know about blood pressure? Tell me what you know about your treatment? What does the rest of your family think? Did you understand what the doctor said?

After discussing the condition of blood pressure and related complications, the consultation should then address the identification of any risk factors. The principal risk factors associated with BP are smoking, excess alcohol intake, lack of exercise and unhealthy diet. Each factor needs to be considered in turn, thoroughly exploring the patient's present habits, in order to negotiate desired goals.

In relation to smoking, there is a need to establish the scale of the present habit and whether this has changed over time. What does the patient understand are the consequences of smoking? Is there a reason why they smoke? Have they ever thought of stopping, and how would they go about it or what goal would they like to achieve? Often specific advice works well. Facts and figures can be important, therefore supplement the consultation with available health education literature.

Consider alcohol in a similar way. Explain how much is an acceptable level (include a diagram of safe levels) and explore ways of coping with reduction where necessary. Help patients set their own goals with ideas such as setting the date to stop smoking; gaining support from family and friends; cutting down alcohol intake and replacing with soft drinks; or not going to the pub so often. Each patient will have different needs and lifestyles, so there is no standard way to approach behavioural modification.

Exercise is another important issue. Does the patient understand the benefits of exercise, and what exercise do they already undertake? What could be realistically achieved? Specific goals will need to be negotiated. The ideal level of exercise is twice weekly for at least 30 minutes and enough to make you breathless.

Finally the patient's diet needs to be considered. Establish what habits the patient has, identifying their likes and dislikes. Determine who does the shopping, cooking and planning of meals, as this will be useful when planning changes. Once again, you need to be realistic. Advise on the dietary benefits of low animal fats, high fibre, low sugar and low salt intake. Emphasize that the diet is not specific to people with high blood pressure, but would benefit the whole family. This will help to establish new dietary patterns. Obviously, if there are specific problems such as obesity or raised cholesterol level a stricter diet may need to be adopted. Very often with dietary control, as with other risk factors, it is useful to include the wife/husband/family in the consultations, in order that the goals may be more readily achieved. Such practice should be encouraged.

Although the consultation will be personalized, it is still essential to recognize external factors which affect patients' behaviour. Society's attitude to smoking has changed radically in recent years and has undoubtedly influenced some people to reduce or cease the habit. Similarly, eating habits are changing, reflected in the increased demand for, and availability of, healthier foods. It is important, therefore, to be constantly aware of what products are available on the local supermarket shelf, to achieve consistently appropriate advice. This also extends to opportunities for exercise and relaxation.

In patients with established risk factors, it may be necessary initially to offer more frequent appointments with the nurse to provide the level of support needed.

Follow-up

Follow-up monitoring is essential to maintain disease control, recognize side effects, avoid complications of disease, and reinforce lifestyle changes. In order for this to be successful the patient needs to understand the need for regular checks and compliance with the recommended treatment. Given the importance of regular review it is essential to have a register of attendance to highlight defaulters, so that necessary action can be taken.

All patients whose blood pressure has previously been raised should receive regular follow-up, whether on treatment or not. This follow-up should consider the undermentioned.

1 *Assessing blood pressure control.* Blood pressures which are elevated but do not need treatment initially may continue to rise until they do. Once treatment is started it must be adjusted until satisfactory control is achieved, which is usually a diastolic BP below 90 mmHg.
2 *Monitoring side effects.* These will only be detected if enquired for. These might include angina, heart failure or renal disease.
3 *Encouraging compliance.* Questions need to be asked about the effectiveness of their treatment and the need to continue with it.
4 *Exclude complications.* These might include angina, heart failure or renal disease.

5 *Risk factor reduction.* Continued attention should be given to helping patients reduce their risk factors. Making significant lifestyle changes is difficult and requires continued support.

The care of patients with hypertension within general practice is undoubtedly developing. Recognition of the nursing role and the establishment of good communication will enable many patients to achieve full compliance with therapy and lifestyle modification. Therein lies good disease control.

References

Beevers, D. G. (1982) Blood pressures that fall on rechecking. *British Medical Journal*, **284**, 71 – 72.

Grimley Evans, J. & Rose, G. (1971) Hypertension, *British Medical Journal*, **27**, 37 – 42.

Hypertension Detection and Follow Up Program Co-operative Group (1979) Five year findings of HDFU program. *Journal of the American Medical Association*, **242**, 2562 – 2571.

Kannel, W. B. (1965) Role of blood pressure in cardiovascular disease; the Framingham Study. *Angiology*, **26**, 1 – 14.

World Health Organization (1978) *Arterial Hypertension*. WHO Technical Report, Series 628.

Further reading

Hawthorne, V. M., Greaves, D. A. & Beevers, D. G. (1974) Blood pressure in a Scottish town. *British Medical Journal*, **3**, 600 – 605.

7 Care of Patients with Diabetes Mellitus

DIABETES mellitus (DM) is a chronic endocrine condition which results in raised blood glucose due to incomplete or absent uptake of blood sugars by the cells of the body. There are two types of primary diabetes—insulin-dependent diabetes mellitus (IDDM), affecting between 1:500 and 1:1000 children under 16; and non-insulin-dependent diabetes mellitus (NIDDM), with a prevalence at around 1% and a peak incidence in the 60s (40 – 50 years in Asians). Secondary diabetes is very uncommon but may be caused by pancreatic destruction (such as following carcinoma or pancreatitis) or insulin antagonism (produced by steroid therapy or pituitary tumours).

The expected number of diabetics in an average practice is eight per 1000 patients with around half on oral agents, a third on insulin and the rest controlled by diet. Each year, a practice might expect to diagnose one new diabetic per 1000 patients.

Presentation

Insulin-dependent diabetes mellitus

This is a fatal condition if untreated. It can occur at any age, but usually presents in adolescence. The cause of IDDM is unknown but it may be an autoimmune reaction against insulin following a viral infection. There is some genetic predisposition, with susceptibility increased by inheritance of HLA DR3 and DR4 antigen tissue types. A child of an insulin-dependent patient has a small (1%) risk of developing IDDM before the age of 20.

Presentation is usually sudden with fairly rapid deterioration, due to the development of ketoacidosis. Presenting symptoms include:

- polydipsia (thirst);
- polyuria (frequency of micturition);
- malaise and lethargy;
- weight loss.

Unrecognized, this can lead to:

- dehydration;
- vomiting;
- severe abdominal pain;
- infection;
- drowsiness or coma.

Non-insulin-dependent diabetes mellitus

This is uncommon in adolescents, with prevalence rising steadily from middle age. By the age of 70 it affects nearly 5% of men and 9% of women. It is frequently associated with obesity (60–90% of cases) and may be precipitated by drug treatment (particularly steroids, diuretics or β-blockers). Although there is familial tendency, HLA types are not associated.

Presentation is normally much more gradual and mild, with symptoms including:

- mild thirst;
- nocturia and polyuria;
- pruritis vulvae or balanitis;
- recurrent boils or furuncles.

Patients may well be asymptomatic and be diagnosed by routine urine examination or following the development of a complication such as:

- cataracts;
- visual loss due to retinopathy;
- resistant infection;
- vascular insufficiency (presenting as leg ulcers, claudication);
- neuropathy (foot ulcers).

Diagnosis

Although diabetes is usually suspected from the finding of a urine test positive for glucose, the diagnosis can only be established by a blood test. High urine sugars can be a normal variant in some patients who are termed high sugar excreters. The diagnosis (of either IDDM or NIDDM) is confirmed by:

1   a single random venous blood sugar of greater than 10 mmol/l; *or*
2   a fasting blood sugar of greater than 6.7 mmol/l.

The corresponding figures for a capillary sample are >11.1 and >6.7 mmol/l. A fasting sugar below 6 mmol/l or random sugar below 8 mmol/l will usually exclude the diagnosis. For the initial diagnosis, the blood specimen should be analysed in a hospital laboratory where quality control is more guaranteed. Subsequent follow-up of blood sugar levels in the practice using blood glucose test sticks (e.g. BM Stix or Dextrostix) is quite appropriate with or without a portable analyser (glucose meter).

In patients with borderline results, a glucose tolerance test can be organized, usually at the local biochemistry laboratory. This involves a fasting blood sugar sample being taken followed by the ingestion of 75 g of glucose in 300 ml of water (1.75 g/kg body weight in children). The blood glucose test is repeated after 2 hours. Patients with an impaired glucose tolerance test, i.e. a venous blood sugar after 2 hours of glucose load between 6.7 and 10 mmol/l, may deteriorate to diabetes in the future (at the rate of 5% per year).

Following diagnosis, an assessment of renal function by serum urea and creatinine is sensible. All diabetics should also receive a serum lipid estimation. Those with abnormal lipids will need very close attention given to dietary modification and close diabetic control. Secondary hyper-triglyceridaemia is associated with poor control. Diabetics with hyper-tension should have baseline electrocardiograms taken.

Health education

This is an essential prerequisite to future good control. As with all health education, it is important to discuss adequately the patient's own fears and beliefs. Information on diabetes should be made relevant to the individual patient. Although better compliance is the goal, the patient should be encouraged and equipped to manage their own disease as far as possible. Follow-up should hope to concentrate on reinforcing positive health behaviour and identifying any disease progression.

Information to cover includes aetiology and the choices for treatment. The benefits of good control should be contrasted with some of the complications of untreated disease. There is accumulating data that the avoidance of long-term complications is linked to good disease control (West 1982). Inevitably it will not be possible to achieve ideal control (fasting sugars below 6 mmol/l and post-meal sugars below 10 mmol/l) in all patients. The age, expectation, ability, compliance, employment and social support of a patient will all need to be balanced against the interference of treatment.

It is very important that advice given in the practice is consistent. This will necessitate adequate involvement of all relelvant parties in developing the practice approach to diabetic care. The most formal approach would be the production of a diabetic protocol. Consistent advice is also achievable through regular discussion between doctors and practice nurses. Other views can be incorporated by involving a local diabetologist, dietitian or diabetic clinic sister. Clinical management topics such as diabetic care are useful motivators to formalize interdisciplinary practice meetings.

Dietary advice

Diet should be as near normal as possible. In fact the best diabetic diet is one that should be encouraged for the whole United Kingdom population, since it is also pertinent to a reduction in cholesterol levels.

Around 50 – 55% of calories should come from carbohydrate, but principally from the more unrefined, complex, polysaccharides (higher roughage foods) including cereals, pulses, pasta, wholemeal bread and potatoes. Refined sugars should be strictly limited. In IDDM the carbohydrate component of the diet is divided into exchanges. Fortunately there is much greater availability of low calorie alternatives today, so that the insulin-dependent child can still drink favourite fizzy drinks and adults may choose a low calorie/low alcohol beer or wine.

Calorie (energy) intake from fats should be reduced from the national average of 42% to around 30 – 35% with the calorie loss made up by high roughage starch. For those patients at higher risk of coronary heart disease or established hyperlipidaemia, this fat should be reduced further to around 25%. At least one-third of fats should be polyunsaturated or mono-unsaturates. This will inevitably involve a shift from dairy products, such as butter and full cream milk to polyunsaturated margarine (if normal weight) or reduced calorie spreads (if obese) and semi- (half-fat) or full-skimmed milk. Meat should be trimmed of visible fat and skin. Cheese should be eaten less frequently with low fat varieties predominating (especially cottage cheese and Edam). Strongly flavoured cheese may encourage the use of smaller amounts. Sunflower and olive oils are recommended; mono-unsaturates like olive oil are particularly worth increasing.

Protein intake should remain unchanged.

Obese patients must be helped to lose weight and obviously their reduction in fat intake should not be compensated for by an increase in carbohydrate calories.

Smoking advice

Support should be offered to diabetics who smoke to help them stop. This is very important as the diabetic has a 100% increased risk of coronary heart disease and a 10% risk of peripheral vascular disease (possibly leading to gangrene and amputation).

Management

The principal aims of diabetic management are listed below. Inevitably there will be the need to balance these aims to suit the indivual patient:

- avoidance of troublesome symptoms;
- elimination of possible causes;

- achievement of good control;
- adoption of healthy lifestyle;
- secondary prevention of diabetic complications;
- minimal disruption to life.

Insulin-dependent diabetes mellitus

Following the diagnosis of IDDM, patients are normally admitted to hospital for stabilization on insulin. The patient will be shown how to give insulin, settled on an insulin regimen, taught the importance of diet self-monitoring, and shown the effects of hypoglycaemia.

In the immediate period following discharge, it is highly desirable that the new diabetic should be seen by the practice team, who will be able to discuss any areas of confusion, reinforce the health education and offer follow-up arrangements in the practice (shared care with the hospital outpatients). At these early visits the nurse should be alert to any sign or symptom of depression as the patient adjusts to the diagnosis.

Diet

Overall principles have been discussed in the section on health education (p. 115). The calories required will be determined by the patient's age, weight and level of activity. The regularity and spread of carbohydrate calories taken throughout the day is more critical in IDDM. This dictates the need for a mid-morning and bedtime snack.

Insulin therapy

For the majority of patients the most appropriate regimen is a subcutaneous injection of an intermediate insulin (usually together with a short-acting insulin) twice daily. A frequent combination is a mixture of soluble insulin and isophane or lente insulin in a 40:60 proportion or fixed dose preparation such as Mixtard. This is then given 20 minutes before breakfast and the evening meal. Insulin therapy should be maintained and possibly increased during illness, even if the patient is not eating much. Doses should be decreased before strenuous exercise or if food intake is reduced. Occasionally a long-acting insulin (such as Ultralente) is used once daily, with regular injections of short-acting insulin, perhaps with a Novo pen, whenever the patient eats. Rarely, a subcutaneous constant infusion of insulin via a syringe driver is used.

Virtually all patients will now use human insulins, 100 iu/ml (U100), which have been developed because they have less antigenicity. This means less insulin need be used and this avoids some of the side effects of treatment. The choice of human insulins is shown in Table 7.1.

Table 7.1 Human insulins.

Preparation	Proprietary name	Manufactuer	Species	Approx. duration of action (hours)	Approx. time of max. effect (hours)	Strength (iu/ml)
Neutral insulin injection	Human Actrapid	Novo	Human	6 – 8	2 – 4	100
	Human Velosulin	Nordisk & Wellcome	Human	6 – 8	2 – 4	100
Mixed insulin (neutral + isophane)	Human Actraphane 30/70	Novo	Human	22 – 24	4 – 10	100
	Human Initard 30/70	Nordisk & Wellcome	Human	22 – 24	4 – 10	100
	Human Mixtard 30/70	Nordisk & Wellcome	Human	22 – 24	4 – 10	100
Isophane insulin injection	Human Insulatard	Nordisk & Wellcome	Human	18 – 24	6 – 12	100
	Human Protaphane	Novo	Human	18 – 24	6 – 12	100
Insulin zinc suspension (mixed)	Human Monotard	Novo	Human	20 – 24	4 – 12	100
Insulin zinc suspension (crystalline)	Human Ultratard	Novo	Human	24 – 36	10 – 12	100

Because these insulins are more potent, patients will usually need to reduce their units when converting from bovine or porcine insulins to human insulin.

Side effects of treatment with insulin therapy

Treatment with insulin may lead to hypersensitivity reactions which can result in rashes or itching. They can be treated by changing to human insulin and antihistamines. Lipodystrophy at the injection site can be improved by using human insulin and rotating where the injections are given.

Insulin resistance occurs through antibody formation, but this rarely affects users of human insulin. Treatment using short courses or steroids might become necessary.

The main side effect to consider is *hypoglycaemia*. This can produce great fear in patients. The symptoms include:

- weakness;
- lethargy, leading to drowsiness;
- tremor;
- paraesthesia (tingling) around the mouth;
- diplopia (double vision);
- slurred speech;
- odd or aggressive behaviour.

Nocturnal hypoglycaemia is suggested by:

- frequent nightmares;
- early morning headaches.

The main signs of hypoglycaemia are:

- pallor;
- sweaty skin.

The diagnosis is confirmed by a blood sugar level below 4 mmol/l. Hypoglycaemia is prevented by good diabetic management, with regular meals and extra carbohydrate after heavy exertion. Patients should know the warning symptoms and always carry some carbohydrate with them. Mild symptoms should respond to 10 g of carbohydrate (three glucose tablets, 2 tablespoons of Lucozade or 2 teaspoons of sugar in a drink). A further 10 g should be taken after 10 minutes if not recovered. For obstructive patients, glycogen 0.5 – 1 mg can be given by subcutaneous, i.m. or i.v. routes. This should relieve symptoms within 20 minutes by mobilizing liver glycogen stores. The dose can be repeated after 20 minutes. Non-responders or patients in a coma should be given 20 – 50 ml of 50% dextrose by i.v. injection.

Non-insulin-dependent diabetes mellitus

The NIDDM patient can be stabilized on therapy in the community. Since they do not develop ketoacidosis there is not the same urgency to bring the blood sugar down. All patients with NIDDM should have a trial of strict dietary control, particularly if they are obese, before considering drug treatment. If their blood sugar is very high (over 20 mmol/l) and they have bad symptoms, the initial reduction of blood sugar levels can be achieved using drugs, but this is rarely necessary. These drugs should then be withdrawn on improvement, to test whether diet alone will maintain control.

Avoiding precipitants

Any possible precipitant should be identified and dealt with. This might be an intercurrent infection. Existing medication which is potentially diabetogenic (for example, steroids, β-blockers, oral contraceptives or diuretics) should be withdrawn or substituted where possible. This may be all that is required to regain control of blood sugar levels.

Diet

The principles have been fully discussed on p. 115. For obese patients a diet of 800 – 1000 kcal (3350 – 4200 kJ) for women and 1000 – 1200 kcal (4200 – 5050 kJ) for men is advisable. This may be increased if weight reduction is achieved.

For the non-obese, calorie intake is normally around 2000 – 2500 kcal (8400 – 10 500 kJ) (200 – 300 g of carbohydrate) in the middle aged or elderly. This will be higher in active younger patients.

Oral drug therapy

If diet is unsuccessful after 4 weeks (8 – 12 weeks in obese patients who are losing weight) then drugs can be added. There are two main types. The main difference between the types is duration of action (see Table 7.2).

1 *Sulphonylureas:* these act by enhancing the patient's existing insulin secretion. They are more potent and have fewer side effects than other oral treatments. For the younger patient, a once daily preparation (like chlorpropamide or glibenclamide) is appropriate. The dose of drug should only be increased every 2 – 4 weeks to avoid accumulation and hypoglycaemia. In the elderly, who are at greater risk of prolonged hypoglycaemia, a short-acting drug should be used (e.g. tolbutamide). This can be dosed 2 – 3 times daily.

Table 7.2   List of oral sulphonylureas.

Drug	Proprietary name	Duration of action	Daily dose		Cost (1989 prices)
			Average	Range	
Chlorpropamide	Diabinese Glymese Melitase	Long	250 mg	100 – 500 mg	< £1.00
Glibenclamide	Daonil Euglucon Libanil Malix	Medium	5 mg	2.5 – 1.5 mg 30 min before meals	< £2 – 3.00
Gliclazide	Diamicron	Medium	800 mg	40 – 80 mg	£3 – 4.00
Gliquidone	Glurenorm	Short	45 mg	45 – 60 mg in divided doses	> £4.00
Glymidine	Gondafon	Short	1 g	500 mg – 1.5 g in one or two doses	> £4.00

In patients with impaired renal function, tolbutamide should be used because of its short action and its elimination by metabolism. Gliquidone appears a safe alternative. Pregnant NIDDM patients should be converted to insulin. In mothers on oral hypoglycaemics there is also a theoretical risk of infant hypoglycaemia with breast-feeding.

The principle side effect of sulphonylureas is hypoglycaemia which can be dangerously prolonged with long-acting drugs. Rashes and blood dyscrasias occur rarely, as can jaundice. Alcohol intolerance (flushing, sweating and tachycardia) can be troublesome especially with chlorpropamide. The antidiuretic effect of chlorpropamide and tolbutamide can produce hyponatraemia (low sodium) and fluid retention.

2 *Biguanides:* metformin (Glucophage) is thought to increase the peripheral utilization of glucose by insulin. It is ineffective in the absence of insulin. It is usually used together with diet and a sulphonylurea in patients who are difficult to control. It is sometimes used as a first line oral agent in obese patients (since sulphonylureas can increase weight).

Metformin should not be used in patients with impaired renal function (since it is excreted by the kidney) or in condition predisposing to lactic acidosis (myocardial infarction, cardiac failure, trauma or liver disease).

Side effects include gastrointestinal effects (anorexia, nausea, vomiting or diarrhoea), lactic acidosis (rare) or malabsorption of vitamin B_{12}.

Insulin therapy

Patients controlled on oral therapy or diet alone may require insulin during pregnancy, infection or illness. Occasionally patients with NIDDM will only be controllable by using insulin, presumably because they have no endogenous production at all. There is no risk of ketoacidosis. The risks and side effects of high blood sugars have to be balanced against the inconvenience of insulin injections.

Complications

Although successful control will avoid the immediate metabolic con-sequences of diabetes (including fatalities), the appearance of complications considerably impairs life expectancy (perhaps by 20 – 30 years) and increases morbidity. Until the introduction of insulin, a young diabetic was fortunate to survive 2 years after diagnosis. Most organs of the body can be affected in the long term, but perhaps the most significant are the vascular complications. In addition, pregnant diabetics are at greater risk of foetal loss or malformation than non-diabetic women. Babies of diabetic mothers are often born larger.

Social and emotional complications are difficult to predict or quantify. However, as with any chronic and potentially debilitating disease, carers should be vigilant to detect psychiatric morbidity and be responsive to any attendant distress.

Ischaemic vessel disease

Macroangiography

Coronary heart disease is doubled, and is a major cause of premature death. Attention to hyperlipidaemia, hypertension and smoking is essential since these all predispose to atherosclerosis (hardening of the arteries) in their own right. Up to 20% of diabetics will suffer a myocardial infarct (Deckert *et al.* 1978). The rate of stroke is also increased with up to 10% of diabetics affected.

Peripheral vascular disease can produce claudication and contribute to chronic foot ulceration. Amputation or gangrene will occur in about 10% of patients. This complication is certainly reduced by good diabetic control (Tchobroutsky 1978).

Microangiography

This is the principal cause of nephropathy and retinopathy, due to damage to the small blood vessels. The actual mechanism is unknown but is, at least partly, related to quality of diabetic control over extended periods. There is also a probable genetic influence which predisposes to microvascular complications.

Nephropathy

Around 40% of young onset IDDM patients will develop renal failure due to diabetic nephropathy. Up to half of these will reach end stage and either die or require dialysis and possibly renal transplantation. Overall, 22% of diabetics develop some uraemia after 25 years of diabetes, rising to 45% after 40 years.

Patients with proteinurea have a 3 – 4-fold excess mortality compared to those with no protein in their urine. Regular follow-up must therefore include a check for albuminuria and hypertension. Once proteinuria is detected, the patient should be followed-up by regular creatinine estimations. Renal function is likely to remain normal for many years. Once it starts to decline it does so progressively, but frequently slowly. When the creatinine is above 200 μmol/l the decline in renal function is inversely linear to the creatinine.

Treatment involves optimal diabetic control. Attendant hypertension should be treated aggressively. There is some evidence that ACE (angiotension-converting enzyme) inhibitors (captopril, lisinopril) are protective of renal function in diabetic hypertensives. Calcium antagonists (nifedipine) or selective β-blockers (atenolol, metoprolol) are also useful, although the latter may compromise oral diabetic drugs or mask the symptoms of hypoglycaemia.

Renal transplantation is the treatment of choice in end stage failure. It becomes necessary when creatinine has reached levels of 700 – 800 mmol/l.

Retinopathy

Diabetic retinopathy is the commonest cause of blindness in the middle-aged, affecting around 10 – 15% of patients. Severe retinopathy changes will be seen in more men (12%) than women (7%). In younger age groups the main problem is proliferative retinopathy with new vessel formation and haemorrhages. Regular (annual) screening by ophthalmoscopy should pick up these problems early when they can be treated by laser photocoagulation, thus preserving vision (Kohner & Barry 1984).

In older patients visual loss is usually due either to macular involvement or to cataract formation. Female diabetics are usually at greater risk of developing cataracts than men (ratio of 6:1).

Background retinopathy

This includes microaneurysms of the capillaries (red dots); large (blot) or small (dot) haemorrhages; hard exudates with yellow rings around leaking capillaries; and maculopathy due to oedema or exudates. These problems do not impair vision unless the macula is involved.

Proliferative retinopathy

Ischaemic changes in the retina promote new vessel formation. If these occur on the disc there is a serious danger of sudden intravenous haemorrhaage and blindness. Although some clearing of the haemorrhage is likely, vision will remain impaired and further bleeds are likely.

Once retinopathy is recognized the annual eye check should be increased to 6-monthly. Maculopathy and proliferative retinopathy require treatment by photocoagulation using an argon laser or xenon arc. This is a painless rapid procedure performed under local anaesthesia. Cataracts, once matured, are treated by extraction with a lens implant or the supply of glasses or contact lenses.

Blindness

Blind diabetics should be registered with the local authority. Special click count syringes (Hypoguard) are available together with audible signal Diastix meters (Hypotest).

Neuropathy

Neuropathy increases with duration of diabetes to affect nearly 50% after 25 years.

Sensory neuropathy

This affects peripheral nerves symmetrically, particularly the legs and feet. The reduction in sensation is often not noticed by patients and can therefore lead to serious damage. Commonly, damage occurs from tight shoes, barefoot walking (on stones, pebble beaches, tacks, etc.) or proximity to fires. Careful patient instruction is needed with regular self-checking.

Painful neuropathy

This is not common but can be extremely severe causing painful paraesthesia (tingling), burning, stabbing pains or skin hypersensitivity. The pain may require strong analgesics, carbamazepine or tricyclic anti-depressants singly or in combination. The pain will always subside after 2 – 3 years and this is important to stress since patients may become suicidal.

Mononeuropathy

This is the sudden loss of function of a single nerve and virtually always resolves spontaneously with no particular treatment. Femoral neuropathy produces pain and wasting of the thigh with loss of the knee jerk. Full recovery occurs within 1 year. Isolated foot drop (popliteal nerve palsy) or carpal tunnel syndrome (median nerve) can occur. Rarely a sudden third or sixth cranial nerve palsy will produce diplopia (double vision) for up to 3 months.

Autonomic neuropathy

Diffuse damage to parasympathetic and sympathetic nerves can occur alongside generalized peripheral neuropathy. This may produce diarrhoea with nocturnal urgency and faecal incontinence. Treatment is with a drug like codeine phosphate or loperamide. Postural hypotension (systolic blood pressure drop of > 30 mmHg on standing) is another sequela. Treatment involves avoidance of hypotensives (sedatives or diuretics) and occasionally the use of fludrocortisone.

Gustatory sweating is a common autonomic neuropathy producing profuse sweating of the scalp, neck and shoulders when eating strong flavoured foods like cheese or curry. Impotence is a common problem in diabetic males, and is usually untreatable. If the patient is continuing to get nocturnal erections with impotence, the problem may be partially psychogenic and referral for psychosexual counselling is appropriate.

Diabetic foot

Neuropathic or vascular complications singly or in combination can produce serious foot problems.

Neuropathic foot

Lack of sensation leads to damage of the skin producing a chronic painless ulcer. These occur mainly over pressure areas where callouses form, especially over the ball of the foot (metatarsal heads) or toes. Trauma may be due to repetitive, or penetrating, injuries or burns. Lack of chiropody care can also cause ulcers. Rest and elevation of the feet is the treatment of choice. Proper footwear is essential, as is a good chiropodist. New shoes should have soft leather uppers and should not be worn for long periods when new. Special shoes should be fitted if any foot deformity exists.

Infection will commonly ensue and this should be promptly treated. If gangrene occurs (particulary toes or foot web) then a local amputation is often successful if the vascular supply is intact.

Ischaemic foot

This produces a painful, cold, pink foot. Pulses in the feet and popliteal fossa are absent. Any ulcer that occurs will be even slower to heal. Patients must stop smoking. Femoral sympathectomy can sometimes stop the pain. Great care should be taken to avoid infection in the foot since, should amputation prove necessary, a local procedure will almost always fail. The higher the amputation that results, the less likely the patient is to maintain independence.

Neuroarthropathy

Loss of sensation together with muscle imbalance may produce unstable, red and painful joints. These Charcot changes are most common at the ankle, metatarsal or metatarsophalangeal joints.

Infections

Vulvitis or balanitis can be treated by clotrimazole cream but will normally settle once the diabetes is controlled. More serious skin infections occur more frequently and may produce a further complication in ulcers secondary to vascular insufficiency or neuropathy. Early recognition and early treatment are essential if damage is to be avoided. Chronic infection of a diabetic foot can be extremely difficult to eradicate without amputation. Antibiotics of choice are flucloxacillin and penicillin (or erythromycin), with metronidazole for deep or resistant infections.

Hyperglycaemia

This acute potential complication in IDDM can be fatal. Uncontrolled diabetics with ketonuria during illness or infection should be treated with increased fluids and frequent injections of short-acting insulin. Patients who are vomiting, drowsy or clinically acidotic should be admitted as emergencies.

Psychological complications

Depression is a possibility. Family or individual counselling may be needed. A psychological cause should be excluded in patients who prove difficult to control, particularly those who swing from hypoglycaemia to hyperglycaemia on a regular basis.

The practice nurse and diabetes mellitus

The practice nurse is ideally situated to be involved in the long-term management and education of patients with diabetes. She will usually be familiar with the family and social background and is therefore in a good position to assess the patient's individual needs. She can also help them to decide on realistic goals to be achieved in diabetic care. If the nurse is full time, continuity of contact is an important factor when problems present outside clinic times. Visits to the home may provide useful information on the home environment and might identify problems with compliance.

A team approach to the care of diabetic patients can work very successfully in the format of a diabetic clinic with a motivated doctor and a practice nurse. Comprehensive health education is important since the disease often presents as part of a syndrome in middle life together with hypertension and hyperlipidaemia with smoking, excess alcohol, lack of exercise and poor diet being frequent associations.

Options for diabetic follow-up in practice

Shared care

Some diabetics will need the additional expert care of the hospital clinics. These include:

- children;
- pregnant diabetics;
- patients with IDDM with progressive complications;
- newly diagnosed IDDM patients;
- patients with NIDDM with poor control or progressive complications.

These patients can be managed by shared care with the general practitioner (GP). An ideal method of ensuring adequate shared care is the provision of a co-operation card. The patient retains the card to attend both the GP and hospital clinic. Continuous documented assessment can be made and investigations will not be duplicated or missed.

The GP mini-clinic

Many diabetics will never need to be referred to hospital. Others may be managed entirely by their own doctor, including:

- most dietary controlled diabetics;
- NIDDM patients without serious complications;
- stable IDDM patients—usually with onset of diabetes after 30 years.

Some of the benefits/disadvantages of the mini-clinic versus hospital clinics are contrasted in Table 7.3.

Table 7.3 Comparison between hospital and GP diabetic clinics.

	Hospital clinics	GP clinic
Attendance	Only 50% attend regularly. 50% defaulters (mainly in ethnic minority groups) are difficult to chase up	Very few defaulters. Defaulters easier to identify and chase up
Appointments	Often long waiting times in crowded and impersonal clinics	Usually no waiting involved. More time can be spent with individual patients
Diabetic control	Good diabetic control for all diabetics	Potentially equally good control
Benefit to patients	Poor continuity of care: patients frequently see a different doctor, although the nurse may be constant	Patient confidence and compliance improved in seeing the same person. Enhances the role of the GP and practice nurse
Screening for other health problems	Not usually done due to lack of time	Easily incorporated into the diabetic clinic

Diabetic care in routine clinics

A separate diabetic clinic within the practice may not be popular with all doctors. Some of the doctors may prefer to look after their own diabetic patients and may be keen to maintain their own clinical skills in diabetes. Patients themselves may wish to see their personal doctor in normal surgery time and these wishes should be respected. Others may not be able to attend a weekly diabetic clinic due to work commitments.

In a practice where there is no formal diabetic clinic, the nurse can still be involved in diabetic care to the same extent, though ensuring regular screening may involve more work. All practices need a filing system (be it card index or computerized) containing diabetic details and a recall date. This enables the nurse to do a monthly search to identify non-attenders.

Patients can be asked to attend 20 minutes early for each appointment with the doctor, so they can be seen first by the nurse. She can perform her screening and educational roles. The patient can then be seen, with the blood sugar result available, by the doctor.

Setting up a diabetic clinic

The following features are needed.

1 *Informed and interested doctor and practice nurse.*
2 *Protected time.*
3 *Method of identifying the patient.* Collecting data for setting up a clinic can be very time consuming and take many months. Involvement of all the staff will be necessary. A special counter book can be used where the receptionists jot down the names of all diabetics that attend the surgery for repeated prescriptions. Many patients' names will be drawn from staff memories. The practice may already have a disease register on a computer with morbidity data recorded, this will make the compilation of a diabetic register much easier.

   All diabetics must be recorded and then categorized into the types: IDDM, NIDDM, and diet-controlled diabetes. The practice nurse should become competent in maintaining diabetic records whether manual or computerized. It would be helpful in the latter system to have a terminal in the nurse's room. Newly diagnosed patients must be added to the list.
4 *Objectives for the clinic.* These might include:
   • educational exercise to motivate patients to adopt appropriate behaviour, e.g. adherence to diet;
   • monitoring of treatment;
   • screening for early detection of complications;
   • prevention of crises;
   • practice protocol for management of diabetics.
5 *A diabetic record card.* This acts as a:
   • check list to maintain good diabetic care;
   • link with the hospital;
   • method to avoid losing important data.

   Various record cards have been devised, some from drug companies. The Birmingham area has devised its own in conjunction with local diabetologists (Figure 7.1). This folds in three to produce a file the size of a Lloyd George envelope. The card is bright fluorescent orange for IDDM diabetics and bright fluorescent green for NIDDM, and is normally carried by the patient until a new one is needed and then stored in the patient's notes.

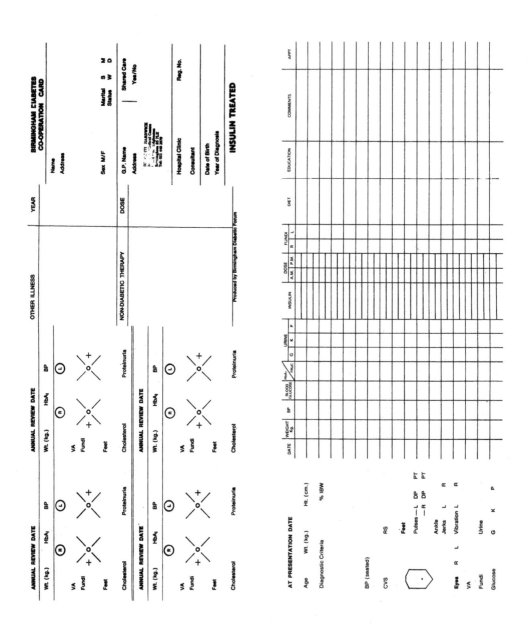

Fig. 7.1 The co-operation card.

6 *Appointment system and follow-up of defaulters.* The frequency of visits to the clinic is variable, dependent on clinical grounds such as compliance and diabetic control. Monthly appointments may be necessary. Once stable, most IDDM patients can be reviewed 3 – 6-monthly and many NIDDM patients can be reviewed annually. The recall data recorded on the computer or diabetic index will enable the practice nurse to follow-up defaulters. This is vital to the successful management of these patients. The nurse can produce a list of all patients overdue for their diabetic appointments at the end of each month.

7 *Support.* Arrangements should be made to have access to the following services, which would be ideally on regular attachment to the practice but if not, should be available for referral:
  • dietitian;
  • local diabetologist;
  • chiropodist;
  • laboratory service;
  • ophthalmologist;
  • educational resources, e.g. district health education department, British Diabetic Association, pharmaceutical companies.

8 *Equipment:*
  • urine testing strips for albumin, ketones, glucose;
  • blood glucose strips;
  • blood glucose meter;
  • lancets or finger-pricking device;
  • scales (preferably ones that can be calibrated);
  • Snellen chart and pinhole;
  • mydriatic drops, e.g. 1% tropicamide;
  • electrocardiograph machine;
  • glaucoma tenometer (optional);
  • cotton wool;
  • sharp object to check for neuropathy;
  • education leaflets;
  • patient monitoring urine/blood record books.

9 *Updating knowledge base.* Continual updating in education for the practice nurse and doctor is vital. Regular meetings of the team involved will provide support and education.

Patient education

The principles of health education in diabetes have been discussed on p. 115. Much practical advice on the disease and its management will also need to be covered. It will not be possible to cover all this in one session with the patient. The order in which the information is shared will depend on the particular needs of the patient, but all the areas should be covered at the same time. Furthermore, it may well be necessary to repeat this education at follow-up appointments.

Initially, the patient may be quite shocked by the diagnosis. Many people have experience of diabetic relatives with serious complications such as blindness, or amputations, so good communication is vital. The nurse should be aware of possible concerns which may not be easily verbalized, by giving information in easy stages and building up a good rapport. This will allow the exchange of learning and teaching.

The first appointment should include a full explanation of the condition, its treatment and implications. Since the IDDM patient will have been stabilized on therapy in hospital already, the priority here is to recap the information provided. This will probably be all the patient can absorb at this session so an appointment for 1 week later can be given, but leave an open invitation for any pressing problem to be discussed. It is useful to tell the patient to jot down a list of questions as they think of them and to bring them along to the next session. Invite a member of the family along to the next appointment and give the patient educational leaflets about diabetes which they can read at leisure.

Dietary advice

Diabetics in the past were encouraged to eat plenty of protein in the form of fat-rich foods such as cheese, and discouraged from eating more than their carefully allotted amount of carbohydrate exchanges. This resulted in an even greater tendency to develop ischaemic heart disease and more premature coronary deaths. The modern diabetic diet is more scientifically valid. The principles are worth reiterating.

1 Reducing the fat content of the diet helps to lower cholesterol (diabetics already have an increased risk of arterial disease).
2 Restriction of high fat protein foods, such as cheese, can reverse microalbuminuria thereby reducing the risk of nephropathy.
3 Fibre in the diet helps to slow down the absorption of sugar from the gut. Several experiments have demonstrated marked flattening of post-prandial blood glucose levels in NIDDM and IDDM when fibre is added to a meal. This is most effective with the glutinous fibre derived from oats, beans and pulses, whereas cereal fibres have less effect. Fibre also has a similar action in lowering blood cholesterol.
4 A complex carbohydrate and increased fibre diet is more filling.
5 Two out of three NIDDM patients are overweight and frequently have poor eating habits. A successful diet may be all they need to treat their

diabetes and often the impact of the diagnosis is enough to change their eating habits (though constant encouragement and support will be needed).

The insulin-dependent diabetic diet

Total energy content of the diet will be worked out, depending on age and lifestyle (a younger, more active patient will need more and an older, less active patient less). The dietary history should be carefully taken and dietary habits disrupted as little as possible. The diet must suit the patient's lifestyle to maintain good compliance. The carbohydrate exchanges will then be evenly distributed throughout the day in a carefully planned diet, and the insulin regimen is worked out accordingly.

The non-insulin-dependent diabetic diet

The nurse has many points to consider when discussing diet with the patient, the most important of all being weight. Is the patient obese? Is a strict calorie-controlled diet necessary? Other considerations include:

- financial—wholemeal bread is more expensive than white, can the patient afford it?
- traditions and food fads (ethics and religious);
- lack of knowledge of healthy foods and how to cook them;
- poor cooking facilities, e.g. no fridge or oven;
- poor shopping facilities—where is the nearest supermarket?
- physical conditions, including failing sight, reduced mobility, anxiety;
- apathy—no interest in changing the habits of a lifetime.

Each patient must be treated as an individual and it is important to educate not only the patient but also the other members of the family. Be realistic about what can be achieved. Weight reduction is the aim in all obese patients. Dietary changes may have to be introduced more slowly; it may take a long time to convert a patient to wholemeal bread!

Dietary advice for diabetic children

Diabetic children's food fads can prove a tremendous problem for their parents. Food refusal can lead to hypoglycaemia and may become a powerful weapon with which to manipulate the parents and medical staff. It is best to advise the parents not to force feed or make an issue out of food refusal. Hunger and low blood sugars will eventually win through and Lucozade or another sugar drink will prevent any major disasters.

Diabetic school children should carry glucose tablets at all times, e.g. dextrosol. School dinners can also create problems as children do not like to be singled out as different, though the new flexible cafeteria-style dinners are better equipped. The British Diabetic Association (BDA) publishes a *Carbohydrate Countdown* to measure the carbohydrate content of food, which is useful for adolescents eating out with their friends. The BDA school pack is useful for a diabetic child and their school teacher in explaining diabetes and hypoglycaemia and how to treat it. Ames Education Services produce a series of 'Rupert Bear and his friends' leaflets aimed at the young diabetic. For non-English speakers, the BDA produces many leaflets on diabetes, ethnic diets, and foot care in various languages including Urdu, Punjabi, Gujerati, Bengali and Hindi.

Specific dietary guidelines for patients are discussed at the end of this chapter in the Appendix (p. 144). This may be of value to practices wishing to produce handouts for their diabetic patients.

Urine testing (glucose and ketones)

There are a variety of urine testing strips all available on prescription, e.g. Diastix, Diabur, Ketostix. The instructions on the bottle must be followed accurately. New diabetics should test urine for glucose until stable, IDDM patients should test before meals and NIDDM patients 2 hours after meals. Once stable, one or two profiles a week at varying times throughout the day before meals is advisable. For good control the urine should be mostly negative, but during illness this may not be so and urine should be tested more frequently.

The IDDM patient should test for ketones using Ketostix when:

- suffering from an infection;
- glucose in urine is >2% for two or more tests in a row;
- blood sugar is raised;
- when eating less than 800 cal (3350 kJ) a day;
- when under stress.

Ketones are chemicals made by the body when it burns fat for energy instead of glucose. If the patient detects ketones they should contact the surgery immediately since diabetic ketoacidosis can lead to diabetic coma.

Blood glucose monitoring

This is a more accurate test and is important for good control particularly:

- pre-conceptually;
- during pregnancy;
- in children;
- during illness to control hyperglycaemia.

Self-blood glucose monitoring must be carried out very accurately and the practice nurse will need to spend time teaching this procedure and observing patient technique. Various glucose strips are available on prescription, e.g. BM Stix, Glucostix. These can be read with or without a glucose meter. Blood monitoring equipment is not prescribable. It should be cleaned and calibrated regularly with frequent quality control carried out by comparing results with laboratory results.

Injection technique

Injection technique will have been taught thoroughly at the hospital but it is important for the practice nurse to be able to reinforce this instruction. Injection sites to recommend are middle or upper thighs, abdomen and buttocks, upper arms and calf (see Figure 7.2). The injection site should be altered regularly so as to avoid lipohypertrophy (lumpiness) and lipo-atrophy (pitting) of the skin. Insulin will not be absorbed properly from these areas.

The insulin is injected by a glass or plastic syringe. Glass syringes are either 0.5 ml with 50 graduations, where one graduation is 1 unit of U100 insulin, or 1 ml with one graduation equivalent to 2 units. The 0.5 inch metal needle of 26 gauge is stored with the syringe in methylated spirit. These should be washed thoroughly once a week. Plastic disposable syringes of 1 ml, with one mark per unit of insulin, are now prescribable. They can be reused several times until the needle is blunt and should be stored in a cool clean place (preferably a fridge) along with the insulin. Insulin should be stored in the bottom of a fridge away from direct heat and sunlight. The expiry date should be checked regularly.

Injecting the insulin is shown in Figure 7.3. When a mixed injection of cloudy and clear insulin is to be given, the clear insulin should be drawn up first, followed by the cloudy using the same method.

Hypoglycaemic and hyperglycaemic attacks

Hypoglycaemic and hyperglycaemic attacks need to be explained carefully. These have been discussed on pp. 119 and 126.

Illness

Instructions for a patient who is ill should include:

- measure blood sugar or urine at least four times a day before each meal;
- if blood sugar or urine is high, increase the insulin or tablets;
- if no food is being taken, it should be replaced by fluid such as milk or Lucozade (one exchange is contained in 50 ml Lucozade, 100 ml of milk or 3 level tablespoons of Complan);
- treatment must never be stopped, either insulin or tablets;
- test urine for ketones in IDDM.

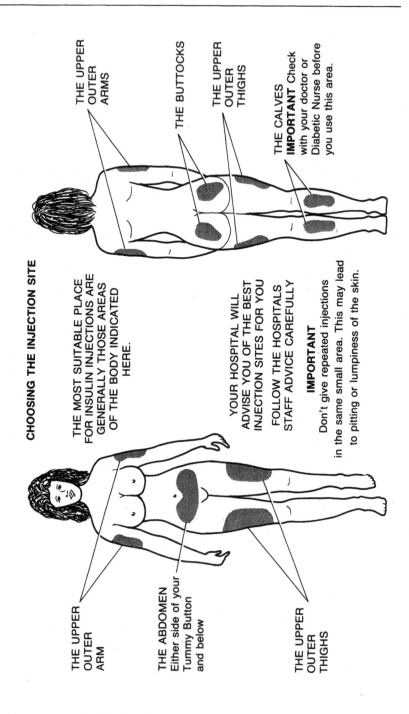

CHOOSING THE INJECTION SITE

THE MOST SUITABLE PLACE FOR INSULIN INJECTIONS ARE GENERALLY THOSE AREAS OF THE BODY INDICATED HERE.

THE UPPER OUTER ARMS

THE BUTTOCKS

THE UPPER OUTER THIGHS

THE CALVES
IMPORTANT Check with your doctor or Diabetic Nurse before you use this area.

YOUR HOSPITAL WILL ADVISE YOU OF THE BEST INJECTION SITES FOR YOU

FOLLOW THE HOSPITALS STAFF ADVICE CAREFULLY

IMPORTANT
Don't give repeated injections in the same small area. This may lead to pitting or lumpiness of the skin.

THE UPPER OUTER ARM

THE ABDOMEN
Either side of your Tummy Button and below

THE UPPER OUTER THIGHS

Fig. 7.2   Recommended injection sites.

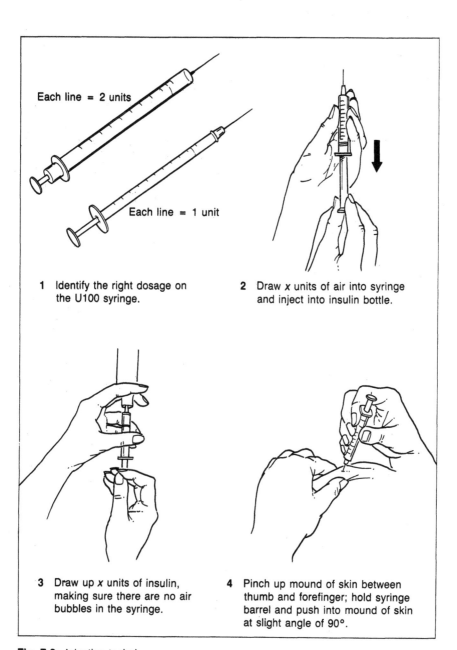

Each line = 2 units

Each line = 1 unit

1 Identify the right dosage on the U100 syringe.

2 Draw x units of air into syringe and inject into insulin bottle.

3 Draw up x units of insulin, making sure there are no air bubbles in the syringe.

4 Pinch up mound of skin between thumb and forefinger; hold syringe barrel and push into mound of skin at slight angle of 90°.

Fig. 7.3 Injection technique.

Diabetic follow-up

This will involve regular checks by the practice nurse and doctor. Patients will perform urine or blood testing. Frequency of testing will be decided by the degree of control, but should be increased during illness. More reliable information is obtained by blood glucose testing. This can be estimated from capillary samples using enzyme strips. Portable glucose meters will read these sticks even more accurately than haphazard testing. Patients should take blood samples before meals on two consecutive days per week since this provides a better indication of overall control than single daily testing. They should know what to do if their blood results are abnormal. In addition, formal assessment of the diabetic should occur at least once a year. This should include the following details.

Height and weight

Do they need to lose weight? Are they losing too much weight? Both are symptoms of poor control and will need to be monitored with regular weighing. Dietary control must be explored, especially fat intake. A target weight should be calculted and aimed for, using the body mass index (BMI). The BMI is calculated from weight (in kilograms) divided by height squared (in metres). A score of between 20 and 25 is the optimum range. Referral to a dietitian may be necessary for particularly difficult cases.

Urine tests

1 Glucose: may signify poor control.
2 Ketones: only necessary if glucose >12 mmol/l. If ketones are present refer to the doctor as the patient will probably need a change in treatment.
3 Albumin: albuminuria in sterile urine may be the earliest sign of nephropathy. Fifty per cent of diabetics develop proteinuria after 30 years of the disease. A mid-stream urine (MSU) test is indicated.

Blood tests

1 Fasting blood glucose. A meter is useful and good technique is essential for accurate results. These results will determine the action that needs to be taken (Table 7.4). Fasting home glucose monitoring is another possibility for the future using blood spots (filter paper). The patient performs the test at home before breakfast and then takes it along to the clinic, thus saving the patient from a long hungry wait at the clinic (Tippletts *et al.* 1989).

2 Glycosylated haemoglobin (HbA_1): taken as 5 ml in EDTA (ethylene-diaminetetraacetic acid) tube, normal range is $5.0 - 8.7\%$; or serum fructosamine: taken as 10 ml in clotted tube, normal range is $2.05 - 2.80\%$.

Table 7.4 Results of fasting blood glucose tests and action which should be taken.

Blood sugar level	Action
<10 mmol/l	No action
10 – 15 mmol/l	Dietary advice with early review
>15mmol/l	May need change in treatment; refer to doctor and reinforce diet

These tests provide information on the state of control over the previous 6 – 8 weeks for HbA_1, and 2 – 4 weeks for fructosamine. Serum fructosamine is becoming popular as it is a less expensive and labour intensive test to perform but a number of studies suggest that HbA_1 is the more reliable measurement (Walford 1989). Other reports have stated recently that fasting blood glucose is as useful and is also much cheaper. These tests rely on the fact that glucose binds to circulating proteins in the blood and the relative concentration of glucose in the blood is reflected by the percentage of proteins that have glucose bound to them. The duration of the test result is dictated by the life span of the particular protein measure (i.e. 6 – 8 weeks for the haemoglobin molecule).

Profile

Particularly important if the patient has repeated albuminuria or hypertension. If the creatinine is raised it is an indication of nephropathy and the patient will need referring to a diabetologist for further investigation.

Fasting lipids

Diabetics have an increased risk of heart disease. Where the cholesterol is greater than 6.5 mmol/l, reinforce the low fat diet and check it 3 months later. If cholesterol is over 7.5 mmol/l and it has not reduced after 6 months of dietary control, than consider referral to a lipid clinic.

Blood pressure

1 Lying: if raised there is an increased risk of heart disease and an increased risk of nephropathy. Follow practice protocol for hypertension.
2 Standing: postural hypotension with a fall in systolic pressure on standing of more than 30 mmHg is a sign of autonomic neuropathy.

Electrocardiogram

This is indicated for patients over 40 years of age, particularly hypertensives.

Eyes

1 *Visual accuity.* Test both eyes using a Snellen chart (and pinhole if refraction is necessary). It is important to have a well-lit room to perform this procedure. The patient must stand at exactly 6 m from the chart with one eye completely covered with opaque card (not with the hand because of the gaps between fingers and blurring of vision afterwards). Reduced visual activity may be a sign of macular oedema. This is invisible on fundoscopy but is important to detect to avoid irreversible central loss of vision.

    The result is recorded as a fraction of six, e.g. if the patient reads down to the bottom line the vision is 6/6 (can read letters at 6 m which should be readable at 6 m). If the patient is unable to read any letters at 6 m they should be registered as partially sighted or blind. For illiterates special charts are used called the E test (the letter E facing different ways).

2 *Dilation of both pupils.* Use a quick acting mydriatic, e.g. 1% tropicamide (can cause stinging of the eyes), which will take approximately 15 minutes to produce full dilation. The patient should be warned that dilation affects the vision for a few hours and driving is not advised. Measuring optic pressures with a tenometer is useful to reduce risks of sudden increase in optic pressures. Any family or previous history of glaucoma should be noted. The patient should be warned to contact the doctor immediately if they get pain, halo vision or marked deterioration of vision following dilation of the pupils.

3 *Fundoscopy.* Performed by the doctor in a darkened room and screens for background established retinopathy and cataracts. If the general practitioner is not performing an annual fundocsocpy, this must be arranged at the hospital diabetic clinic or with an ophthalmologist. Problems identified in general practice should preferably be referred to an ophthalmologist with an interest in the diabetic eye.

Feet

Close examination of the feet is very important. Simple scrutiny, palpation, using of a tuning fork, pin and cotton wool are all that is needed. Signs of neuropathy to exclude are:

- absent temperature impulse;
- absent touch impulse;

- absent vibration;
- abnormal motor effects (or absent jerks);
- increased blood flow;
- unnoticed trauma from ill-fitting shoes, nails or stones;
- burns from hot water bottles or sitting too near the fire;
- plantar ulcer, caused by callous, friction or pressure;
- Charcot foot, deformity of bones in foot following injury;
- neuropathic oedema leading to ulceration;
- claw toes due to muscle wasting caused by neuropathy.

Signs of ischaemia to exclude are:

- no pulses palpable (popliteal, posterior, tibeal, dorsalis pedis);
- pain;
- pink feet and hairless legs;
- cold feet;
- ulcers, usually found at the points of frequent trauma;
- infection, with discharge, swelling and throbbing.

Assessment should also include:

- skin atrophy (thickening and cracks in the soles of the foot);
- need for chirpody (ingrowing toe nails, callouses, subungual ulceration);
- need for orthopaedic assessment (retracting toes, bony prominences).

Education of the patient regarding foot care is essential. Instruction to the patient should include the following list:

- examine your feet daily;
- wash your feet daily (avoiding hot water) and dry thoroughly especially between the toes; if vision is impaired, personal nail cutting should not be attempted;
- consult a chiropodist;
- keep the skin supple with a moisturising cream;
- never walk barefoot indoors or outdoors;
- do not put feet on hot water bottles or too close to a fire;
- always wear proper fitted shoes with a wide fitting insole for cushioning;
- examine your shoes daily for cracks, pebbles, etc. which may not be felt if you have a loss of sensation;
- cover minor cuts with a sterile dressing.

Diabetic patients can receive free National Health Service chiropody care and should have ingrown nails, corns and callouses treated by chiropodists. Supplies of wide fitting shoes can be ordered by mail order catalogue from Cooper Footline Ltd, Sycamore Works, Tilton on the Hill, Leicestershire LE7 9L9. When ordering, draw around the feet and send this to the suppliers. Peter Lord and the 'Ecco' range of shoes also do a wide fitting range and these are available in a number of department stores.

Additional follow-up

The practice nurse can assess the self-monitoring techniques and reinforce any teaching. The importance of avoiding diabetic complications and coronary risk factors must be stressed. Help with lifestyle modification may be needed:

- do they smoke? If so, how many? Is there a smoking cessation clinic in the practice?
- how many units of alcohol do they drink per week? (maximum safe allowable is 12 units/week in men and 9 units/week in women);
- do they know that alcohol intoxication mimics the signs of hypoglycaemia?
- diet, obesity, low fat, high fibre content must be reinforced;
- can the whole family be involved in positive lifestyle change to encourage compliance?

Other screening

The nurse can also take the opportunity to offer other screening facilities such as cervical cytology and breast checks. Flu vaccines can also be offered.

Doctor follow-up

The doctor at the initial and annual visit will work with the nurse, performing some of these tasks. Particular responsibilities will include:

- physical examination;
- fundoscopy;
- treatment decisions.

Special advice

Pre-conceptual advice

Diabetic control must be optimized for several months before pregnancy. Diabetic women should be assessed for complications, particularly hypertension, renal disease or ischaemic heart disease. Those women controlled on oral therapy should be advised about insulin injections which will be needed during pregnancy. Stopping smoking is essential.

Contraception

The progesterone-only pill followed by sterilization when the family is complete is the most reliable form of contraception for diabetics. There is no additional risk of vascular disease with progesterone, and this does not affect carbohydrate metabolism. Barrier methods like the diaphragm, IUCD (intrauterine contraceptive device), and the Depo-Provera injection are useful alternative methods. The combined pill is contraindicated in diabetes.

Driving licences

Once the DVLC has the patient's application form they write to the doctor direct for information about their diabetic control. The driving licence will be issued for 1, 2 or 3 years and renewals made free of charge. The patient should not drive if:

1 there are any eyesight problems (vision below 6/16) or loss of sensation in limbs;
2 they have difficulty recognizing early symptoms of hypoglycaemia which may affect their judgement;
3 they are being stabilized on insulin (until stabilization is complete).

At the first sign of hypoglycaemia the diabetic driver should stop the car, take carbohydrate and then leave the car until the symptoms have disappeared. This is to make it clear that they are no longer in charge of the car. Unfortunately, they could be charged with driving under the influence of drugs or without due care. For more information contact the British Diabetic Association.

Insurance

It is very important to declare diabetes on applications for insurance purposes. Again it usually results in a supplementary form for the doctor's attention. Although it will probably result in an increased premium or regular medical, the result of non-disclosure will be that the insurer will not pay for any claims. The British Diabetic Association pamphlet DH134 outlines these facts in more detail.

Nurse education

It is important that all members of the team are well informed and clinically up-to-date in the care of diabetes. Additional training for the practice nurse is essential before setting up a diabetic clinic. The various options include the following.

1 Diabetes study days such as those organized by the British Diabetic Association (BDA) or at local hospitals.

2   Practice nurse courses which include diabetes in their programme.
3   In-service training at hospital diabetic clinics. Diabetic liaison sisters are usually willing to let nurses sit in at the clinic. Contact the consultant personally to explain your reasons for attending, or ask the doctor to help with an attachment.
4   Postgraduate journals including *Balance* (BDA journal); *Practical Diabetes*; *Pulse*; *The Practitioner*, etc.
5   Some pharmaceutical companies offer training facilities. Ames hold diabetic study weekends (Miles Laboratories Ltd, Stoke Court, Stoke Poges, Slough SL2 4LY, Tel. 02814 5151). Servier Laboratories produce a *Guidelines for Practice Nurses* pack (Servier Laboratories Ltd, Fulmer Hall, Windmill Road, Fulmer, Slough SL3 6HH, Tel. 0753 662744).

Appendix: The diabetic diet—guidelines for the patient

Eat fibre-containing foods

Increase amounts eaten of wholemeal bread, crispbreads and biscuits, and wholegrain cereals, e.g. Weetabix, Bran Flakes, Shredded Wheat, porridge. Eat more brown rice, wholemeal pasta and spaghetti, wholemeal flour, potatoes, fruit and vegetables. Use lentils or dried beans in stews to replace some of the meat, e.g. butter beans, red kidney beans, chick peas.

Eat less fatty foods

Use skimmed milk (or semi-skimmed if the patient cannot accept skimmed) instead of whole milk. Grill, roast, stew or boil instead of frying. Cut off fat from meat and skin from chicken. Use less butter, lard or margarine. Change to a polyunsaturated margarine (or calorie-reduced margarine if obese). Fatty foods to avoid are chips, roast potatoes, fry ups, pâté, mayonnaise, crisps, cream and pastry.

Avoid sugar and foods containing sugar

Glucose, jam, marmalade, honey, syrup, treacle, chocolates, sweets, cakes, cream, tinned fruit in syrup, puddings made with sugar, condensed milk, evaporated milk, fruit squash, and fizzy drinks, Ribena and Lucozade should all be resisted. Use sugar-free squash and fizzy drinks, e.g. Diet Coke. Have drinks without sugar or use sweeteners, e.g. Canderel.

Do not drink alcohol on an empty stomach or in large quantities

All alcoholic drinks are fattening whether they contain sugar or not (Table 7.5). If you are overweight you should avoid all alcohol. Furthermore the following should be noted.

1 With diabetic tablets, smaller quantities of alcohol make you drunk (tablets and alcohol interact with each other).
2 If you are taking chlorpropamide, alcohol may cause severe facial flushing.
3 Some low sugar beers and ciders have a higher alcohol content.
4 Avoid sweet wines, sweet vermouth and all liqueurs except brandy or absinthe.

Table 7.5 Carbohydrate (CHO) content of popular drinks.

0.5 pint ordinary bitter	= 180 cal	(750 J)	= 10 g CHO	= 1 exchange
1 pint lager	= 180 cal	(750 J)	= 10 g CHO	= 1 exchange
0.75 pint stout	= 220 cal	(925 J)	= 10 g CHO	= 1 exchange
1 pint dry cider	= 200 cal	(850 J)	= 10 g CHO	= 1 exchange
5 pub measures extra dry Martini	= 80 cal	(335 J)	= 10 g CHO	= 1 exchange
1 pub measure Dubonnet	= 106 cal	(450 J)	= 10 g CHO	= 1 exchange

Wines vary according to their sweetness. Spirits (whisky, gin, vodka) contain no or very little sugar and may be allowed in moderation. Do not buy diabetic beers or other food products; these brands are unnecessary, very expensive and can cause diarrhoea if drunk to excess due to the high sorbitol content.

Salt

Use only a small amount in cooking and do not add at the table. Try using herbs and spices in its place. Liberal use of ground black pepper is safe and can help high salt users to reduce their consumption.

Additional guidelines for the overweight NIDDM patient

Follow the diabetic diet as above, but eat fewer calories.

1 Eat plenty of vegetables and salad (avoid oily dressings and salad cream).
2 Eat only lean meat and cook without added fat or oil. Drain off fat from casseroles or roasts.
3 Avoid fatty meat products, e.g. pâté, sausages, luncheon meat.

4 Have fish or poultry at least three times a week (about 125 – 150 g poultry or 175 – 200 g fish with each meal).
5 Use skimmed milk in drinks, on cereals and in cooking.
6 Use cheese very sparingly and preferably use low fat cheese such as cottage cheese, Edam or Camembert.
7 Have fruit at least once a day.
8 Have a target weight and be weighed as often as needed for motivation, maybe even once a week.

Religious and ethnic aspects of diet

Some people follow a religious culture very strictly and this must be respected when educating about a diabetic diet.

Hinduism

Many Hindus are vegetarian and do not eat meat, fish, eggs or anything made with them. The cow is particularly sacred. Alcohol is forbidden. Fasting is also part of their culture and the adviser must be aware of this. Although religious rules will allow people to avoid fasts on medical grounds, some patients will still wish to observe them. This would not be advisable for IDDM patients, but sufferers of NIDDM can be advised on how to prepare for fasts safely. Adequate fluid intake is essential, as is reduced activity.

Sikhism

An offshoot of Hinduism with similar dietary restrictions.

Muslims

Pork or pork products are banned and so is alcohol. During Ramadan there is no eating or drinking between dawn and sunset.

The Asian diet

The Asian diet has plenty of fibre in the form of vegetables, pulses and beans and therefore has many good points. The problem with the diet is the high fat content, e.g. ghee, which is used in most of the cooking. The patient should be advised that cooking without oil is successful. Only 2 teaspoons of oil, ghee or butter is acceptable per day. One medium chapatti (thin) is equal to one slice of bread from a large loaf, which is equal to 2 tablespoons of rice. In a calorie-controlled diet, only three chapattis per day are allowed. Foods to avoid include bhajjia, samosa, potato vadai, chevora, sev, gantia, papri, puri, crisps, cream, tinned milk, salad cream and mayonnaise. Also avoid sugary foods including jaggery, sugar, jam, honey, jalebi, gulab, jama, sikand, peda and barfi. Poor cereals are scero, semya, kneer and cakes.

Appendix: Useful addresses

The British Diabetic Association (BDA)

10 Queen Anne Street
London W1M 0BC
Tel. 01-323 1531

As well as what has already been mentioned, they offer holidays for 5 – 15-year-olds; eight activity courses for 13 – 25-year-olds; family weekends throughout the United Kingdom; and advice for carers.

Information Folder on Diabetes

Royal College of General Practitioners
14 Princes Gate
Hyde Park
London SW7 1PU
Tel: 01-581 3232

Diabetic Medicine (journal of the BDA)

Journals Department
John Wiley & Sons Ltd
Baffins Lane
Chichester
Sussex PO19 1UD

Practical Diabetes

The Newbourne Group
Greater London House
Hampstead Road
London NW1 7QQ

References

Deckert, T., Roulsen, J. E. & Larsen, M, (1978) Prognosis of diabetics with diabetes onset before the age of thirty one. *Diabetologia*, **14**, 371–377.

Kohner, E. M. & Barry, P. J. (1984) Prevention of blindness in diabetic retinopathy. *Diabetologia*, **26**, 163–179.

Tchobroutsky, G. (1978) Relation of diabetic control to the development of microvascular complications. *Diabetologia*, **15**, 143–152.

Tippetts, A., Callaway, P., Leatherdale, B. & Rowe, D. (1989) Assessing glycaemic control of NIDDM: acceptability of blood sampling at home. *British Medical Journal*, **298**, 497–498.

Walford, S. (1989) Monitoring in the diabetic clinic. *Practical Diabetes*, **6**(2), 56–58.

West, K. M. (1982) In *Complications of Diabetes*, 2nd edn., (ed H. Keen & R. J. Jarrett). Edward Arnold, London.

Further reading

Bradshaw, C. A. (1989) A protocol for nurse-run diabetic clinics in general practice. *Practical Diabetes*, **6**(2), 70–71.

Crabbe, M. J. C. (1987) *Diabetic Complications: Scientific and Clinical Aspects*. Churchill Livingstone, Edinburgh.

Day, J. L., Humphreys, H. Davies, H. (1987) Problems of comprehensive shared diabetes care. *British Medical Journal*, **294**, 1590.

Faris, I. (1982) *The Management of the Diabetic Foot*. Churchill Livingstone, Edinburgh.

Kinson, J. & Nattrass, M. (1984) *Caring for the Diabetic Patient*. Churchill Livingstone, Edinburgh.

Mann, J. (Oxford Diabetic Group) (1982) *The Diabetes Diet Book*. Martin Dunitz, London.

Paul, A. A. & Southgate, D. A. T. (1978) *The Composition of Foods*. HMSO, London.

Royal College of General Practitioners (1988) *Information Folder on Diabetes*. RCGP., London.

Royal College of Nursing (1989) *Diabetes—Clinical Guidelines for Practice Nurses*. Royal College of Nursing, London.

Simpson, H. (1987) Diet for diabetics—a critical review. *Practitioner*, **231**, 1450–1454.

Watkins, P. J. (1983) *ABC of Diabetes*. BMJ Publications, London.

8 First Aid and Emergencies

THIS chapter may seem superfluous to a book principally discussing an extended role for nurses. Treatment room duties may be seen as the most mundane, traditional and least professionally developing role in the practice nurse workload. However, emergency treatment can be a stimulating and stressful part of clinic work and does promote problem solving skills. Any health professional who is ill prepared for the patient who suddenly collapses or suffers a severe allergic reaction could compromise reasonable standards of care.

First aid is defined as the immediate care given to a person who has been injured or has been suddenly taken ill. This can be further divided into life-threatening or acute immediate care situations. In life-threatening situations, first aid can mean the difference between life or death, temporary or permanent disability, and rapid recovery or long hospitalization. Indeed, everyone in the health service, from porters to administrators, should be capable of attempting resuscitation on a collapsed person. Unfortunately training on this important, but rarely needed, skill is sadly lacking, even amongst doctors.

There have been many studies demonstrating that cardiopulmonary resuscitation (CPR) increases survival rates in patients with ventricular fibrillation who receive CPR within 4 minutes; or defibrillation, intubation and i.v. fluids within 8 minutes of cardiac arrest. Because ventricular fibrillation occurs in 55 – 60% of people with cardiac arrest, prompt CPR is important. Since heart disease is the biggest killer in this country, cardiac arrest has been the most frequently studied situation in relation to life-threatening first aid treatment.

In general practice a potentially iatrogenic (medically induced) cause of cardiac or respiratory arrest could be anaphylactic shock, secondary to injections such as routine immunizations or antibiotics. Other dramatic life-threatening situations might include severe bleeding, major burns, head and spinal injuries, internal injuries, musculoskeletal injuries, drowning or shock.

Inevitably some of these are dealt with first in hospital casualties. However, it is important that practice nurses are prepared for these infrequent, but life-threatening medical emergencies. They should consider attending a Red Cross First Aid course to learn how to do CPR and other first aid procedures correctly and effectively: supervised hands-on practice is needed for competence in future unexpected emergencies. Further information can be obtained from the local British Red Cross Society or by telephoning the London main office (01-235 3241).

This chapter will focus on acute immediate care situations most likely to present in the general practitioner's surgery. It should help a practice nurse to deliver competent, safe and appropriate care with a physician on or off the premises. At a minimum, it should identify deficiencies in acute care skills which require further training. However, it must be stressed that although all nurses should be knowledgable on the methods of diagnosing and managing emergencies, to be actually involved in regular use of these skills with patients requires certain minimum criteria. These include practical and documented training, written practice agreements on what the nurse can perform on her own and arrangements for back up. This will be an area for negotiation in individual practices. The point at which referral to the doctor is needed must be clearly stated.

Taking a history

With any presenting emergency other than cardiac arrest, there are key symptoms and history that must be ascertained. When all these questions are answered the nurse will have a basis on which to provide nursing care.

1   The patient's age.
2   Description of events surrounding onset:
    • any event occurring with onset?
    • has there ever been a similar episode in the past?
    • was the onset sudden or gradual?
    • what was the duration, is it still present?
3   Location of illness/injury.
4   Description of symptoms, such as quality of pain:
    • ache;
    • burning;
    • sharp;
    • dull;
    • constant;
    • intermittent;
    • is it radiating? Has the pain moved?

For example, coronary pain may radiate to the jaw, or appendicitis may begin as periumbilical pain.

5   What precipitated the symptom? What seems to make it worse?
6   What helps, or relieves, the pain? What has been tried?
7   If it has occurred in the past:
    • when, where, how many times?

- what investigations have been done and with what results?
- results of past treatment?
- past diagnoses?
- pattern of symptom: same, worse, or better?
8 Effect on activities of daily living?
9 Why is the patient here now? Why is he or she seeking help now?
10 Does the patient have his or her own ideas or beliefs about what the problem is?

Cardiac arrest

The principle behind treating cardiac arrest is to maintain cardiorespiratory function artificially until the patient regains his or her own heartbeat and adequate respiration, and/or can be transferred to hospital. Cardiac arrest is frequently unexpected, although it usually occurs in people with acute or chronic cardiac or respiratory disease. Cardiac arrest (syncope) may be the first symptom of cardiac disease for up to one-third of coronary heart disease (CHD). Signs of cardiac syncope include absent pulses and blood pressure, unconsciousness, absent or gasping respirations, and cyanosis.

Cardiopulmonary resuscitation

Before starting CPR, another member of staff should be alerted to telephone 999 and then assist in resuscitation. The basics of CPR are as follows.

1 Establish an airway:
- examine the throat for foreign objects, remove if present; this includes dentures;
- insert an airway. Make sure the tongue is forward. If an airway is not immediately handy the tongue can be elevated by moving the jaw forward;
- begin assisted respiration. The practice treatment room should always have an airway and Ambu bag;
- if possible, attach oxygen to the Ambu bag;
- secretions in the throat may need suctioning.
2 Cardiac massage:
- put patient on hard surface. Either place a board behind his or her back or place patient on the floor;
- position the heels of the hands on the lower third of the sternum. The movement will be of a rocking nature with the weight of the body used to compress the heart between the sternum and the spinal column;
- the patient should receive two breaths initially;

- check the pulses;
- if alone, cardiac massage should be two breaths to 15 compressions;
- if two people are available, then one breath to five compressions at the rate of one compression per second should be used.

3 If a cardiac monitor or electrocardiograph (ECG) and defibrillator are available a trace should be taken. Defibrillation may be indicated and could be life-saving.
4 An intravenous line should be available in the treatment room for establishing acute drugs if the nurse is qualified for inserting it, or a doctor is available. A 5% dextrose solution is ideal. Insert the cannula along a long bone (the radius is a good site) to ensure stability of the needle.
5 Once initiated, CPR must continue until the patient recovers, the rescuer is exhausted, or the patient is pronounced dead.
6 Make accurate records after the completion of CPR.

Open wounds, suturing and dressings

Basic assessment for wound care should include determination of bacterial contamination and extent of tissue damage. Ideally, wounds should be repaired within 6 – 12 hours but, with debridement and antibiotics, facial wounds can be closed after 12 hours to minimize scarring. There may be other factors that can complicate wound healing, such as diabetes, vascular disease, poor hygiene, malnutrition or non-compliance. Check whether tetanus immunization is up-to-date.

Generally, wounds caused by bites, especially human and cat bites, have high bacterial counts and should therefore be left open to heal. The exception might be for wounds on the face where close observation and antibiotics should be considered. Cats have long thin teeth and carry *Pasteurella multocida*, so co-trimoxazole or tetracycline should be used. Dog bites need to be carefully evaluated but may not need anti-biotic cover, depending on the site, depth and confidence in patient compliance.

A significant amount of hand laceration may occur during fighting. A careful history is needed and documentation is a must. As the object causing the laceration can determine the proper treatment and follow-up, this must be identified and noted.

Cleaning

Effective cleaning of all wounds must include washing with soap or antibacterial skin cleanser (such as povidone-iodine solution) which does not harm exposed tissues, followed by irrigation with normal saline or water. This will remove contaminated matter, micro-organisms, some necrotic tissue and provides some debridement. Cotton wool is less irritating than gauze, but cotton wool fibres can stick in the wound. The slight abrasiveness of gauze can help to dislodge contaminants.

A syringe with or without a needle can be used to irrigate wounds. All visible contaminants such as dirt, gravel or glass must be removed to minimize scarring or infection and to prevent tattooing. Solutions such as alcohol, hydrogen peroxide, Eusol and others have been found to be leukocytic, i.e. to destroy the white cells necessary for healing. The correct technique in cleaning wounds is more important than relying on antibiotic coverage to prevent infection. Minor wounds can be cleansed during daily bathing with any mild soap (some perfumed soaps may be irritating and could possibly cause allergic reactions).

Suturing

If the wound is large, or on a joint, or must be closed for cosmetic reasons, sutures may be necessary. Sutures are more precise than Steri-Strips. If anaesthesia is going to be used, lignocaine with adrenaline is better than plain lignocaine because the duration is longer and will help to minimize bleeding.

- If using lignocaine, be sure that nerves and tendons are intact before anaesthesia and wound closure.
- Do not inject more than 20 ml lignocaine in order to avoid a systemic reaction.

The patient will find it less painful to have the lignocaine injected into the edges of the wound rather than through intact skin.

There are two suture types: absorbable and non-absorbable. Dexon is absorbable and is dissolved by autolytic action, rather than phagocytosis as with the older gut types. This helps to minimize the inflammatory response. This suture is strong and has a long life of 90 – 120 days.

Of the non-absorbable, synthetic sutures, the braided type is preferable, such as Surgilon or Ethibond. Because these are synthetic there is less tissue reaction and they can be left in place longer. The advantage of braided sutures is that they are reputed to be easier to handle. Monofilament, synthetic sutures such as Ethilon and Prolene have the advantage that monofilament is believed to result in less tissue reaction than braided sutures.

On the face, 5-0 or 6-0 width sutures should be used; on the trunk and extremities, 4-0 and 5-0 should be used. When suturing the skin there must not be too much tension since there will be continued swelling for

48 – 72 hours after an injury, thus increasing the tightness of the sutures. Extreme tension contributes to the railroad appearance of scars. There must also be great care to approximate the skin edges to the wound.

Sutures on the face should be removed earlier than on the rest of the body. Facial sutures should be removed after 3 – 4 days, although scalp wounds should be left up to 10 – 14 days. On the rest of the body sutures are removed 5 – 10 days after suturing.

Dressings

Dressings should fit the wound. A minor, dry wound may be left open to the air after washing with soap and water. A dry dressing of gauze or Melolin may absorb some discharge, as long as the surrounding tissues are basically healthy and intact. These dressings should be secure, but not air tight.

Open unepithelized tissue requires moist dressings such as Granuflex. This may stay on the wound for as long as 4 days to allow healing without daily wound disruption at dressing changes. Synthetic plastic dressings such as Tegaderm are indicated for wounds without profuse discharge, such as first or second degree burns or unopened decubitus ulcers. This is used as a 'second skin'. Abrasions can be treated similarly to burns because of the loss of skin. Topical antibiotics should not be used since these can cause sensitization or allergic reaction.

If packaging of a large wound is necessary, tight packing keeps the wound open and impedes healing. The packing should therefore be loose to promote closure. If damp packing is required Dakin's solution can be used, 0.2% saline, 0.2 – 0.5% hypochlorite solution, or (for a *Pseudomonas* infected wound) use 0.5% acetic acid. A wet dressing will need to be changed before it is allowed to dry out. This may require at least one daily dressing changes.

Wounds will continue to discharge and swell for up to 48 hours. After 24 – 48 hours there is usually a fibrin seal which seals the wound from bacteria. At this time it is safe to gently clean the wound. Continued dressings are likely to provide protection from external trauma, rather than soak up tissue discharge.

Careful instruction to the patient should help to maximize wound healing and prevent complications.

1   The wound should be kept clean and dry.
2   If the dressing becomes wet it should be changed.
3   The patient must return to surgery if there is:
   - redness;
   - swelling;
   - increased pain;
   - increased discharge.

4 Pain and swelling can be reduced by elevating the injured area by:
- sleeping on extra pillows;
- resting a limb on a chair or table.
5 Warn the patient that some extra swelling may occur after exercise.
6 An injury is a weakened area, so try to avoid re-injury.
7 Activities may need to be limited.
8 Avoid the sun to prevent irregular pigmentation on new skin formation.
9 Mild pain should respond to paracetamol or aspirin.

Overdose

There are several considerations for first aid following ingestion overdose, both accidental and intentional. Many people who have overdosed will need follow-up at hospital, but what can a nurse do in the surgery if alone or if the ambulance is delayed? With an unconscious patient, the maintenance of an airway will be the most important consideration; however, the more likely presentation in the surgery is a conscious patient.

Some ingestions, including pills, need to be eliminated through emesis. It would be dangerous, however, to induce vomiting of other ingestions, such as oil-based products like petroleum (which may occur when mouth siphoning petrol) and some pesticides or fertilizers. If there is any aspiration during emesis of these substances, the resultant chemical pneumonia can be fatal. If there is ingestion of acid or base solutions, there is burning during ingestion and should emesis be attempted there will be burning of the tissues again.

To induce emesis, syrup of ipecacuanha can be used. It can empty the stomach for up to 12 hours after ingestion. This is because there is often a delay in gastric emptying, especially if a drug that slows gastric motility has been taken. In remote areas where medical care is likely to be delayed, a family with small children should be encouraged to have syrup of ipecacuanha alongside their paracetamol since accidental ingestions are not uncommon for small children, especially when exploring homes or visitor's handbags. The peak years for accidental overdoses in children are between 1 and 4 years old. The quicker the vomiting occurs, the less poison is absorbed. Ipecacuanha doses are 10 – 15 ml for children and 30 ml for adults followed with liquids. Warm liquids seem to cause vomiting quicker than chilled drinks. The purpose is to get as much fluid down as possible, so any clear liquid will do, but water is generally the quickest and easiest. The dose of ipecacuanha may be repeated after 15 – 20 minutes if there is no response.

Because of the multitude of ingestibles it is sensible to telephone the local casualty department for management advice prior to treatment. Sometimes water only is advised, the rationale being to dilute the poison. Do not give milk because it could stimulate a chemical reaction in the stomach with further burning and damage. In this instance, care needs to be taken to avoid giving so much water that the patient gets nauseous and vomits.

If the exact dose and nature of ingestion is known, after consulting with casualty there may be no need for further treatment. If follow-up at the hospital is needed to determine toxicity, transportation should be arranged. If the patient can go home, the casualty officer may suggest activated charcoal to be taken 2 hours after ipecacuanha. The rationale for charcoal is that it binds the drug in the intestinal tract. Unfortunately it is difficult to administer and stains if the patient vomits. If passed in nappies it will stain everything it comes in contact with. It is, however, very safe to use.

Enema may be considered, but would be contraindicated in the absence of bowel sounds, intestinal obstruction or electrolyte imbalance.

If there has been an intentional overdose psychiatric care is imperative. Always suspect that overdoses are intentional if they occur in children of 8 or 9 years old. Childhood depression and suicide does occur. Accidental overdoses may frequently be managed in the general practitioner's surgery, but only after consultation with the doctor or casualty department.

There are many ingestions that cause patients great concern such as money, bugs or buttons. Generally, as long as the object has been swallowed and there is no respiratory distress and no sensation of foreign body in the oesophagus it will be expelled in the stool. However, one ingestion that needs hospital advice is the swallowing of small batteries. The gastric juices can corrode batteries, releasing poisonous acid. It is always better to be safe and refer these to the casualty department for management.

Should any information on the management of poisoning or overdoses be required, specialist advice is always available at the following poison control centres. Contact the nearest to you for up-to-date information on all drugs, chemicals or poisons, including their identification, prognosis and acute or chronic treatment. All are manned 24 hours per day.

- Belfast Royal Victoria Infirmary (0232-240503);
- Birmingham Dudley Road Hospital (021 554 3801);
- Bristol Royal Infirmary (0272-230000);
- Cardiff Royal Infirmary (0222-709901);
- Dublin Poisons Information Centre, Beaumont Street Hospital (0001 – 379964/379966);
- Edinburgh Royal Infirmary (031-229 6907);
- Leeds General Infirmary (0532-432799);
- London Guy's Hospital (01-407 7600/01-635 9141);
- Newcastle Royal Victoria Infirmary (091 2325131).

Seizures / convulsions / fits

Seizures can be frightening to see and cause much anxiety to observers. However, most seizures are self-limiting and will stop on their own. Ensure that the airway is clear; the simplest way is to roll the patient on to his or her side and remove false teeth if possible. Check that the patient is in a safe place. The floor in the waiting room may well be safer than an examination table away from constant observation. Do not push anything into the mouth, in case there is soft tissue injury to the gums or even a broken tooth. If a seizure is prolonged, that is lasting more than 15 minutes, a doctor will be needed for possible drug therapy. Fitting for less time poses absolutely no threat to health. Think of possible causes of seizures to ensure proper treatment.

- Is this a known epileptic?
- If so, has medication been taken?
- Is this the usual seizure pattern?

This person will most likely only need observation. Medical decisions will be made by the doctor.

- Is this person a diabetic and in hypoglycaemic shock?

In this case the nurse should have a dextrose solution ready for intravenous injection.

- Is there an untreated infection such as meningitis?
- If a baby is seizuring, what is the temperature?

A febrile baby can be sponged down, allowing the evaporation of the water to bring down the body temperature.

If a seizure is prolonged the doctor may elect to use intravenous diazepam, 5 – 10 mg for an adult. However an easier option to administer is rectal diazepam available as a special formulation like a mini-enema (Stelozid rectal tubes). These are available in dosages of 5 mg (children) or 10 mg (adults) and can be repeated after 15 minutes when necessary. In cases of certain epileptic seizure (known history or accompanying relative/friend) it would be safe for a practice nurse to administer one dose of rectal diazepam if a doctor were not immediately available or whilst awaiting an ambulance, ideally this would be included in practice nurse protocols. Prolonged fitting (greater than 20 – 30 minutes) can be associated with brain anoxia and damage, or cause troublesome future epilepsy. A decision to treat should therefore be urgently considered after 15 minutes have passed. A description of the seizure, where it began, how long it lasted and where it spread is usefully recorded. Ultimately, the doctor must make decisions regarding follow-up.

Some seizures can be reduced by education, particularly correct medication regimens. Does the diabetic person know symptoms of impending hypoglycaemia and what to do? Can they do instant blood testing? Does the epileptic person know how to take his or her medication properly and return for proper follow-up? Some babies have a lower seizure threshold for febrile seizures. Do the parents know how to recognize a fever and what to do about it? Generally, it is the rapid rise in temperature that triggers the seizure. This peak from normal to high within a few hours does not allow the body to acclimatize to the higher temperature. A parent who has a baby who is seizure prone must be alert for sudden febrile illness which may reduce fever, and should treat the child quickly with an antipyretic (paracetamol syrup) and tepid sponging.

> Remember, do not give aspirin to children under the age of 12 years due to the rare but devastating Reye's syndrome.

Frightening as seizures can be to all concerned, the primary first aid is nursing care to the patient and reassurance to the onlookers. Once the convulsion is over, known epileptics can be advised to rest (or sleep if drowsiness is a feature) at home. Admission is not necessary if the seizure was uncomplicated, however the patient must be assessed by a doctor before a final decision is made. Recurrent attacks should, however, prompt a review of medication. First convulsions, especially in children, should be admitted for assessment. In addition, children with a prolonged fit, no obvious source for a fever, and a persisting neurological deficit should also be admitted. Meningitis can present with a convulsion and may be difficult to clinically diagnose in young children.

Red eyes

An eye injury or infection is a fairly common presentation in the general practitioner's surgery. It is important to differentiate between a minor, easily attended eye injury, and a serious disorder that may threaten vision. A careful history must be taken, which describes the onset of the problem and the past history. Some key questions should identify possible visual changes, pain or severity, itching, crusting on waking, tear production, discharge, photophobia, and if there is a sensation of a foreign body. If there has been an injury, note the incident details carefully. Could a foreign body have entered with high velocity, e.g. chips from a hammer? Is the foreign body possibly iron? If there are chemical burns, note the name of the substance. If there has been a blow to the eye, was the force a minor bump or was it powerful? Be careful about penetrating wounds that seem innocuous. For instance, rose thorns can carry fungus that can be very difficult to treat.

Referral to an ophthalmologist for careful assessment is mandatory for:

- a distorted pupil;
- a tear of the iris (iris will not be round);
- hyphaema;
- marginal laceration;
- lacrimal duct damage;
- any suspicion of a penetrating wound;
- suspicion of iritis;
- corneal laceration (though not an abrasion);
- acute vision loss;
- any unusual eye problem.

After an accurate history, a careful examination must be done. For baseline and medico-legal reasons, a visual acuity must be done and documented. Bear in mind, though, that normal visual acuity does not exclude possibly serious eye injury.

The eyelids must be examined. Are they healthy? If not, describe them. Some oedema is common in allergies or after much rubbing. Is there an obvious stye? Examine the conjunctiva and sclera. Check the distribution of redness; redness that extends into the iris could indicate iritis.

Examine the iris, pupil and anterior chamber. The iris should be clear, without redness. The pupils and iris should be round. Examine the pupils and the reaction to light—both pupils should be the same size and should react equally. The anterior chamber should be clear.

A crude measurement of peripheral vision can be done by checking the visual fields by confrontation. The nurse should face the patient and the patient should cover one eye. The patient should stare at the nurse's nose. While flicking a finger the nurse should slowly bring her arm into the midline from an extended position. The patient is instructed to say when the moving fingers can be seen in the corner of his or her vision. This check is done from at least four areas: from above, below and each side. It is then repeated on the opposite eye. If there is any finding of loss of peripheral vision the general practitioner must be notified.

Eye problems cause much concern for health care providers, therefore if in any doubt, consult with a doctor. Two basic rules for the prescription of drugs for eyes are as follows.

1 Do not send the patient home with topical anaesthesia. Pain is common with many eye problems and anaesthesia could mask a serious problem. If the pain is severe or is getting worse the patient needs another examination. Pain should be managed with oral analgesia, cool packs to the eye, and a patch to stop the blink reflex which may be irritating.

2   Do not use steroids without an ophthalmological opinion. Steroids can impede the immune system so any infection, particularly viruses (such as herpes simplex which produces dendritic ulcers), could worsen. This could possibly result in a corneal ulcer perforating.

Most of the eye problems discussed so far should also be assessed by the doctor. However some of the following presentations can be safely seen by a suitably trained nurse after an appropriate eye examination.

Allergic conjunctivitis

This may occur suddenly, usually after exposure to an allergen such as cats, pollens, grasses or cigarette smoke. There may be conjunctival swelling, itching, red eyes, clear discharge or profuse tears. Generally this is more common during allergy seasons and is accompanied by other atopic symptoms such as runny nose, sneezing or itching.

Try to identify the allergen for future avoidance. Many people may find bathing and washing their hair will help to wash away the allergen. Cool compresses may alleviate the swelling. Allergic conjunctivitis is self-limiting (will get better on its own), but if medication is prescribed Opticrom eye drops is a good first choice drug. This helps prevent re-occurrences and may need to be used regularly during the allergy season.

Bacterial conjunctivitis

Generally, the discharge is purulent rather than clear as in allergic reactions. If the conjunctivitis is mild it can be treated with cool compresses for the discomfort, and the discharge cleaned with boiled water and cotton wool balls. Remind the patient that the infection can spread from eye to eye if good hygiene is not observed. Remind women that they can spread or re-infect themselves with contaminated make-up, such as mascara wands. If a prescription is necessary, chloramphenicol drops or ointment can be used.

Foreign bodies

Only diagnose a foreign body if there is a very clear history, such as 'I think I have an eyelash in my eye'; 'I can't find my contact lens'; 'I was sanding and now have dust in my eye'; or 'the wind blew something into my eye'.

Often the foreign body will be visible. The safest way to remove a foreign body is irrigation. Large quantities are needed so connect up an i.v. bag of normal saline with tubing and use this to rinse out the eye. A sterile syringe without a needle and sterile saline could also be used for irrigation, but carefully and gently. Another way is to wet a cotton wool bud with sterile water or saline and then very gently remove the object. A dry cotton wool bud is irritating and increases the risk of causing a corneal abrasion. If a foreign body cannot be seen evert the upper eyelid over an orange stick. If there is nothing to be seen but there is still the sensation of a foreign body, use fluorescein paper and a Wood's lamp. This will fluoresce a corneal abrasion which can mimic the sensation of a foreign body.

Once a foreign body is removed, or corneal abrasion is identified, chloramphenicol eye ointment may be used after consultation with a physician. Additionally, an eyepatch will help to stop the blinking reflex which could cause continuing discomfort for the patient. Most minor corneal abrasions heal spontaneously within 24 hours. In all cases of corneal abrasion a physician should be consulted.

Eye problems can be serious. If the nurse's examination does not elicit a clear diagnosis and the nurse is even slightly unsure, the patient needs further evaluation. When in doubt, consult.

Head injuries

These may include bumps on the head or lacerations. Assessment can be difficult and careful evaluation, examination and follow-up is extremely important. First, take an accurate history. Consider the following:

- did the patient have a seizure and then fall?
- did the patient faint and fall?
- what was the force of the blow?
- was the injury observed?
- could drugs or alcohol complicate your examination?

Danger signs that indicate further evaluation is absolutely necessary, either by the doctor or preferably referral to hospital, include:

- prolonged amnesia or unconsciousness at site;
- depressed level of response;
- neurological abnormality on arrival;
- clinical or X-ray evidence of fracture;
- fits, vomiting or severe headache.

When in doubt, *always* consult.

The neurological examination must include:

1 *Blood pressure and pulse:* remember your paediatric cuff for children.
2 *Mental status:* is the patient orientated? Ask for today's date, day of the week and time of the day. Is the patient alert and aware of his or her surroundings? Can they completely describe the injury, before and

after? Is the patient acting 'normally'? Does the injury involve a very small, preverbal child? Does the child have an adequate historian?

3 Examination of the cranial nerves:

I   olfactory (generally not checked);
II   optic—visual acuity; look for papilloedema in the fundus;
III   oculomotor—papillary reactions to light and accommodation;
IV   trochlear—test extraocular movements;
V   trigeminal—palpate temporal and masseter muscles;
VI   abducens—check for nystagmus; check facial sensations; corneal reflex;
VII   facial—notice any weakness or asymmetry; raise eyebrows; frown; close eyes tightly; show teeth; smile; puff out cheeks;
VIII   acoustic—assess hearing;
IX   glossopharyngeal—check for hoarseness;
X   vagus—check for hoarseness; check soft palate and uvula by having the patient say 'ah'; the palate and uvula should stay even, without unequal rising or the uvula pulling to one side;
XI   spinal assessory—shrug shoulders against examiner; push cheek against examiner;
XII   hypoglossal—inspect tongue (should be able to move tongue from side to side).

4 *Examination of the motor system:* is the patient's walk sure and balanced? Carry out Romberg's test: have the patient stand with feet together and eyes closed, and stand close in case the patient loses balance. Loss of balance could indicate cerebellar disease. Does the patient have equal grips?

5 *The sensory system:* is there numbness? Is sensation symmetrical?

6 *Reflexes:* these should be present symmetrically.

If after an examination you feel the injury is minor and that the patient can go home it is important that a responsible adult is present. Head injuries can quickly become life-threatening. The instructions to the responsible adult should include:

1 Wake every hour for the first 6 hours after injury and assess arousability or level of consciousness. The patient may sleep, but must be roused hourly.

2 Check that all four extremities are moving.

3 Give no drugs that may alter consciousness, such as alcohol or tranquillizers.

4 To treat pain give paracetamol only; do not give aspirin because of blood-clotting interference.

5 The patient must telephone or return if he or she vomits more than once, the level of consciousness decreases, the pain increases, or any symptom occurs that concerns the carer.

The nurse *must* document the history, examination, assessment and instructions given.

Anaphylaxis

Anaphylaxis is a dramatic hypersensitivity reaction that usually occurs within seconds to minutes after an exposure to an allergen. The most common iatrogenic anaphylaxis is a reaction to an injection, either immunizations or antibiotics. **All general practitioner surgeries should have adrenaline 1:1000 readily available during immunization clinics.** Every patient should wait in the waiting room for 15 minutes after any injections. Desensitization injections are associated with a particular risk of producing anaphylaxis and are not now recommended for use in the community. They should not be offered without full resuscitation facilities. Some people are also allergic to local anaesthetics. Anaphylaxis may also occur after insect bites, especially from bees, wasps and hornets.

The presentation of anaphylaxis may be hives or urticaria, and wheezing. The patient can quickly progress to cyanosis, shock and unconsciousness. Treatment must be immediate. Adrenaline 1:1000 will be needed immediately. Prefilled syringes can be ordered for the surgery from the local chemist. The dose is 0.05 ml (3 – 5 months); 0.07 ml (6 – 11 months); 0.1 ml (1 year); with the maximum paediatric dose 0.3 ml; adults 0.3 – 0.5 ml. This may need to be repeated after 5 – 10 minutes. The patient may need oxygen because of hypotension and upper airway oedema. An airway should always be available. Ideally the nurse will have received resuscitation training.

If the allergen is in an extremity, such as an injection or insect bite, use a tourniquet to slow venous return from the site but do not cut off the arterial supply. Keep the extremity below the level of the heart. Apply cold to the site of the sting.

Such a patient will need transport to the hospital as soon as possible, but must receive immediate first aid. Because of possible impending shock an indwelling intravenous catheter should, where possible, be inserted prior to transport to allow for i.v. treatment in case of circulatory collapse (when veins would become very difficult to find).

The patient must be subsequently contacted for complete health education. They must know their allergen so they can notify future health care providers. Their file must be clearly marked. If the patient had a reaction to shellfish he or she may also have an allergy to the dyes used in X-ray studies. The patient should be informed about this possible link. The patient should also be advised to wear a Medic Alert tag.

A patient who is allergic to insects should be advised not to run barefoot on grass. They must also be informed how to minimize the amount of venom expressed by the insect. When stung by a bee, scrape the bee off, do not pick the bee off as the squeezing action can squeeze more venom into the body. If a patient is likely to be at risk, such as a farmer ploughing isolated fields, the patient should have his or her own prefilled syringe with adrenaline with careful instructions on its use.

Nurses working in isolated agricultural areas or anywhere a doctor may not be readily available, should have a clearly written protocol about anaphylactic shock. Because of possible anaphylaxis, immunizations and injections should not be given without a physician and adrenaline on the premises.

Appendix: First aid/emergency drugs

The following list is only a guide. Compare this to your own supplies. Consider using this list as a basis for discussion at a practice meeting or local nurses group.

1   *Cardiac – respiratory – diuretic:*

Adrenaline 1:1000 0.5 ml ampoules available in prefilled syringes.
Aminophylline 250 mg in 10 ml ampoules. *Caution:* too much, too fast leads to tachycardia, cardiac irregularities; or seizures that do not stop until drug wears off. *Ideally* given slowly while on cardiac monitor.
Hydrocortisone 100 mg vials.
Lignocaine hydrochloride 2% in 20 ml vials.
Frusemide 20 mg in 2 ml ampoules; or bumetanide 2 mg in 1 mg vials.
Nifedipine 10 mg in 2 ml. Used for supraventricular tachycardias.
Glyceryl trinitrate 0.5 mg (or Nitrolingual spray).
Ventolin inhaler/nebulizer.

2   *Analgesics:*

Morphine sulphate 20 mg. Can also be used for pulmonary oedema.
Pethidine 100 mg in 2 ml.
Paracetamol 500 mg tablets.
Lignocaine 2% with or without ephedrine.

3   *Antibiotics:*

Benzylpenicillin (Crystapen injection) 300 mg per vial. Dose depends upon age and weight.

4   *Emetics* (for accidental ingestions/overdoses):

Ipecacuanha emetic mixture for paediatrics: 6 – 18 months 10 ml; 18 months – 10 years 15 ml; adults 30 ml.
Activated charcoal.

5 *Sedatives:*

Diazepam 10 mg in 2 ml.
Haloperidol 5 mg in 1 ml.

6 *Antidotes:*

Naloxone (Narcan) 0.4 mg in 1 ml.

7 *Diabetic:*

Dextrose injection 50% in 50 ml ampoules.
Insulin.
Glucagon injection.

8 *Ophthalmic:*

Fluorescein paper.
Chloramphenicol drops or ointment.

Further reading

American Red Cross (1981) *Standard First Aid and Personal Safety.* Doubleday & Co., New York.

Bates, B. (1983) *A Guide to Physical Examination.* J. B. Lippincott, Philadelphia.

Cope, A. R., Quinton, D. N., Dove, A. F., Sloan, J. P. & Dave, S. H. (1987) Survival from cardiac arrest in the accident and emergency department. *Journal of the Royal Society of Medicine,* 80(112), 746 – 749.

de la Roche, M. R. P. (1987) Is prehospital advanced life support really necessary? *Canadian Medical Association Journal,* 137(11), 995 – 999.

Elkington, A. R. & Khaw, P. T. (1988) The red eye. *British Medical Journal,* 296, 1720 – 1724.

Elkington, A. R. & Khaw, P. T. (1988) Injuries to the eye. *British Medical Journal,* 297, 122 – 125.

Finley, J. M. & McConnell, R. Y. (1984) *Emergency Wound Repair.* University Park Press, Baltimore.

Goroll, A. H., May, L. & Mulley, A.G. (1981) *Primary Care Medicine.* J. B. Lippincott, Philadelphia.

Heimbach, D. M., Hunt, T. K. & Rauscher, G. E. (1987) Suiting the dressing to the wound. *Patient Care,* 21(11), 164 – 176.

Hoole, A. J., Grennberg, R. A. & Pickard Jr., A. G. (1982) *Patient Care Guidelines for Nurse Practitioners.* Little, Brown & Co., Boston.

Hutchison, J. H. & Cockburn, F. (1986) *Practical Paediatric Problems.* Lloyd-Luke Medical Books, London.

Mills, K., Morton, R. & Page, G. (1984) *A Colour Atlas of Accidents and Emergencies*. Wolfe Publications, London.

Rakes, R. E. (1988) *Conn's Current Therapy*. W. B. Saunders & Co., Philadelphia.

Rosman, N. P. (1987) Emergency pediatric head trauma. *Patient Care*, **21**(11), 192 – 216.

Wasson, J., Walsh, B. T., Tompkins, R. & Sox Jr, H. (1975) *The Common Symptom Guide*. McGraw-Hill, St Louis.

Wilson, D. H. & Marsden, A. K. (1982) *Care of the Acutely Ill and Injured*. John Wiley & Sons, Chichester.

9   The Way Forward

IT would be irresponsible to make assumptions as to how practice nursing will develop in the future. However, there are certain trends emerging which may point the way. The principal trend is the work being developed on preventing disease and the care of people with chronic diseases. In both fields of care, nursing has a particular contribution to make because of the requirement for a continuing long-term involvement with clients which often has relatively little need for medical input. We mentioned in the Preface that primary health care is changing, and becoming more orientated towards these activities, and it is easy to see why nursing has become involved. Work in disease prevention is likely to become a bigger priority for practices following the proposed contractual changes (Department of Health 1989), although it is to be hoped that this will not be at the expense of other areas of care. There will be great pressure to reach targets on immunizations and smears if cutbacks are to be avoided. Nurses will have to be participants in this work, otherwise there will not be the manpower to do it, or maybe even the will. It is not always easy to keep up enthusiasm for anticipatory care, and nurse involvement may make it more interesting and more manageable.

There is also a likelihood in the future that general practitioner employers will have to ensure that practice nurses are properly educated for the job. It will become compulsory for them to be educated specifically for this role, and to be properly updated from time to time. This education should be reimbursable.

Practice nurse education has been the subject of much debate since the publication of the Cumberledge Report (Department of Health & Social Security 1986). This report states that practice nurses have little educational preparation for their work and have been taught procedures by doctors rather than nurses. The debate continues and indeed has been raised during the joint preparation of this book. What is without doubt is that practice nursing is seen as a distinct speciality with its own skills and priorities.

Many practice nurses have a considerable amount of experience and expertise in their work, but few have much in the way of post-registration qualifications (Cater & Hawthorne 1988; Greenfield et al. 1989). One could argue that this does not matter, and in many ways it does not, as long as the work is done safely. However, there is value in acquiring recognized experience and expertise if they contribute to academic respectability and to income. It seems likely that a system of continuing education may soon be introduced for nurses in which educational units can be accredited by completing courses or attending conferences. Such units may be used either towards another qualification (for example, a degree) or for compulsory annual updating of knowledge. If this system is adopted, it would seem to be an excellent way for practice nurses to prove their worth to the wider nursing profession, and to themselves as a group of specialists. It is also desirable for practice nurses to become tutors, so that in-service support and tuition is available for the novice.

It is interesting to note that in the United States, when the first nurse practitioners were trained, they were taught by doctors. Eventually, there were sufficient nurse practitioners with enough experience to become tutors themselves, and the courses are now headed by nurses. It is inevitable that with so much overlap in skills and knowledge, doctors will need to be involved in the initial stages of practice nurse education. However, when there are enough practice nurse tutors, nurses should provide their own education. If practice nurses and doctors are working together as teachers then educational priorities can enhance teamwork.

Linked to this educational attainment is the importance of building a research base to underpin practice nursing. Why has practice nursing developed? What is its value to clients and patients? What sort of education level is necessary for its practice? These questions have yet to be answered, because so little is known about the nature and value of practice nursing. Most of the outcome studies available are from the United States and should be augmented by British studies. Research studies on both the process and outcome of practice nursing will become more common, and a research base will evolve.

There are exciting times ahead for pratice nursing as it develops. This burgeoning nursing speciality requires and deserves continuing educational opportunities and its own body of literature. Like many branches of nursing its value has not been thoroughly understood and, perhaps, its potential for improving primary health care has not yet been achieved. With our lack of impact on the major causes of morbidity and mortality, with the advances in knowledge about anticipatory care, and at a time of great uncertainty for the National Health Service, the practice nurse's contribution to primary care is more necessary than it has ever been.

References

Cater, L. & Hawthorne, P. (1988) *The Nurse in Family Practice*. Sintari Press, London.

Department of Health & Social Security (1986) *Neighbourhood Nursing: A Focus for Care*. Report of the community nursing review, HMSO, London.

Department of Health (1989) *General Practice in the National Health Service. The 1990 Contract*. HMSO, London.

Greenfield, S. M., Stilwell, B. & Drury, V. W. M. (1987) Practice nurses: social and occupational characteristics. *Journal of the Royal College of General Practitioners*, **37**, 341 – 345.

Index

ACE inhibitors (*see* angiotensin-converting enzyme inhibitors)
Aerolin Autohaler 76–7
age and hypertension 93
alcohol intake
    and diabetes mellitus 145
    and hypertension 93, 98
allergic conjunctivitis 160
allergies and asthma 68
alpha-receptors 92
alveoli 66
aminophylline 73
anaphylaxis 163–4
ancillary staff 16, 19
    numbers of 47
    salary reimbursement 15
    see also primary care team
angina and hypertension 94
angiotensin 92
angiotensin-converting enzyme (ACE) inhibitors 100, 123
antenatal clinics 20
anticholinergic drugs 72
anticipatory care 24–5, 47–62
antihypertensive drugs 98–100
arteries, effect of hypertension on 94
Asian diet in diabetes mellitus 146–7
assertiveness 42–3
asthma 65–89
    diagnosis 68–71
    extrinsic/intrinsic 67
    improving care 85
    occupational 68
    organizations 88–9
    patient education 84
    role of practice nurse 85–7
    symptoms 68
    treatment 71–5
        delivery systems 75–84
        trigger factors 67–8
Asthma Society Training Centre 88
atenolol 99
atheroma and hypertension 94
Atrovent 72
attached staff 20–1
    see also primary care team audit 23–4
    cervical cytology screening 60
    hypertension protocol 102
    and screening clinics 54, 61
autonomic neuropathy in diabetes mellitus 125

background retinopathy 124
balanitis 126
baroreceptors 92
basic practice allowance 14
beclomethasone (Becloforte, Becotide) 74
bendrofluazide 99
Berotec 72
beta-blockers 99, 123
beta-receptors 92
beta$_2$-stimulants 72
biguanides 121
bites 152
blindness in diabetes mellitus 124
blood glucose monitoring 134–5, 138–9
blood pressure
    in diabetes mellitus 139
    measurement 96, 105
    physiology 92–3
    see also hypertension
bodily contact 31–2
body language 28, 29, 31–2
body mass index (BMI) 138
brain, effects of hypertension 94
Bricanyl 72
British Diabetic Association 147
bronchial hyperreactivity 67
bronchioles 66
bronchodilators 72–3
budesonide 74

calcium antagonists 99–100, 123
cancer, opportunistic screening for 52
capitation fees 14–15
captopril 100
cardiac arrest 151–2
cardiopulmonary resuscitation (CPR) 149, 151–2
carpal tunnel syndrome 125
case finding 25, 105
cataract in diabetes mellitus 124
cerebral haemorrhage and hypertension 94
chest X-ray in asthma 72
chiropody care in diabetes mellitus 141
chlorpropamide 120, 121
codes of speech 29, 30
communication skills 27–45
community nurses 20
community psychiatric nurses (CPNs) 20
conjunctivitis 160

consultation, tasks for   34–41
continence services   21
contraception in diabetes mellitus   142–3
convulsions   157–8
coronary heart disease in diabetes
  mellitus   122
  mortality rate   49, 50
  prevention project   53–62
  screening for   51
    opportunisitic   52
corticosteroids   73–4
  trial of   69
Cumberledge Report   6–7, 20, 167

delegation to practice nurses   1–2
depression in diabetes mellitus   127
diabetes mellitus (DM)   113
  care options   127–9
  clinics   128, 129–31
  complications   122–7
  diagnosis   114–15
  diet   116, 117, 120, 132–4, 144–7
  follow-up   138–43
  health education   115–16, 131–7
  management   116–22
  nurse education   143–4
  organizations   147
  presentations   113–14
  record card   129, 130
  role of practice nurse   127
  secondary   113
diabetic foot   125–6
Diabetic Medicine   147
diet
  in diabetes mellitus   116, 117, 120,
  132–4, 144–7
  and hypertension   98
dietitians   21
diplopia   125
disease mortalities   49, 50
Diskhaler   80
District Health Authority (DHA)   11–12
District Unit General Manager,
  involvement in team meetings   22
dressings   154
driving and diabetes mellitus   143
drugs in first aid   164–5
dry powder devices   80–2
Duovent   75

electrocardiography in diabetes
  mellitus   140
emergency nursing   149–64
  drugs   164–5
emesis   155
empathy   39–40
enalapril   100
equipment checking   56

Executive Council   12
exercise
  and hypertension   98
  test   70
external controllers   34
eyes
  examination in diabetes mellitus   140
  injury/infection   158–61

facial expression   31
Family Practitioner Committee (FPC)   12
fasting blood glucose   138, 139
fasting lipids   139
febrile convulsions   157, 158
feeling good about oneself   42–5
feet, in diabetes mellitus   125–6, 140–1
femoral neuropathy   125
fenoterol   72
first aid   149–64
  drugs   164–5
fits   157–8
foreign bodies, ocular   160–1
Friends of the Asthma Research
  Council   89
fundoscopy in diabetes mellitus   140

general practice   11
  changes in structure   12–14
  financing   14–16
  provisions of NHS Act   12
general practitioners (GPs)
  delegation to practice nurses   1–2
  vocational training   14
gestures   31, 32
glibenclamide   120, 121
gliclazide   121
gliquidone   121
glucose tolerance test   115
glycosylated haemoglobin (HbA),   139
glymidine   121
group practice   12, 13
gustatory sweating   125

haematuria in hypertension   95
haemoglobin estimation in asthma   71
head injuries   161–2
health, concepts of   33–4
health education   28, 48
  in asthma   84
  in diabetes mellitus   115–16, 131–7,
  144–7
health motivation   33
health promotion   24, 47–62
health summary cards   56, 57–8
health understanding   33–4
  exploration of   35–6
health visitors   20
heart, effect of hypertension   94

helping relationship 39–41
helping skills, developing 41–2
heredity and hypertension 93
Hindu diet in diabetes mellitus 146
history-taking 34–5
    in emergencies 150–1
hormone replacement therapy and
    hypertension 93
human insulins 117, 118
hydrochlorthiazide 99
hyperglycaemia 126
hypersensitivity reactions 163–4
hypertension 91
    consequences 94–5
    definition 91–2
    follow-up 110–11
    initial consultation 108–10
    malignant 94
    organization of care 101
    patient assessment 96–7
    protocol 59–60, 101–6
    record card 102, 103–4
    as a risk factor 95
    risk factors for 93, 106
    role of practice nurse 100–1, 107–8
    secondary 93
    significance 95
    treatment 98–100
        decision to start 97–8
hypoglycaemia 119, 121

illness
    concepts of 33–4
    and diabetes mellitus 135
impotence 125
infections in diabetes mellitus 126
information, presentation of 37–8
ingestion overdose 155–6
inhalation therapy 76–84
inhaled steroids 75
injection technique in diabetes
    mellitus 135, 136, 137
insulin-dependent diabetes mellitus
    (IDDM)
    diagnosis 114–15
    diet 133
    management 117–19
    presentation 113
    see also diabetes mellitus
insulin therapy 117–19
    in non-insulin-dependent diabetes
        mellitus 122
    side-effects 119
insurance and diabetes mellitus 143
Intal 74
internal controllers 34
ipratropium bromide 72

ischaemic vessel disease in diabetes
    mellitus 122–3, 126
items of service fees 15

jargon 37

ketones 134
ketotifen 74
kidney
    effect of diabetes mellitus on 123
    effect of hypertension on 95

left ventricular hypertrophy and
    hypertension 94
lifestyle, alteration of 48–9
lipoatrophy 135
lipodystrophy 119
lipohypertrophy 135
Local Medical Committee (LMC) 12
locus of control 33–4
log book 60

maculopathy in diabetes mellitus 124
marriage guidance services 21
Medical Practices Committee (MPC) 12
medical secretaries 19
metered dose inhalers 76
metformin 121
methylxanthines 73
midwives 20
mononeuropathy in diabetes mellitus 125
morning dip 69
'MOT' clinics 53–62
Muslim diet in diabetes mellitus 146
myocardial infarction
    and diabetes mellitus 122
    and hypertension 91

National Asthma Campaign 89
National Health Services (NHS)
    expenditure on 16, 17, 18
    general practice budget in 15–16
    structure 11–14
National Health Service Act 1946 11, 12
Nebuhaler 79–80
nebulizer 83–4
nedocromil 74
negotiation 38
neuropathy in diabetes mellitus 124–5,
    126
nifedipine 99
non-insulin-dependent diabetes mellitus
    (NIDDM) 113
    diagnosis 114–15
    diet 133, 145–6
    management 120
    presentation 114
    see also diabetes mellitus

non-steroidal anti-inflammatory drugs and
  hypertension 93
non-verbal communication 28, 29, 31–2
Nuelin 73
nurse practitioner 2, 168
  in British general practice 3
  comparison with practice nurse 3–4
  contribution to patient care 5–6

occupational therapist 21
opportunistic screening 25, 51–2
  see also screening
oral contraceptives and hypertension 93
orthoptists 21
overdose 155–6
Oxford Prevention of Heart Attack and
  Stroke Project 53–62

paraesthesia in diabetes mellitus 125
parentcraft classes 20
patients as clients 48
peak expiratory flow rate (PEFR) 68–9
  home monitoring 70
  specific tests with 69–70
peak flow meter 68–9
  home use 70
  tests using 69–70
peripheral vascular disease 122
personal appearance 31
personal space 32
persuasive communication 38–9
Phyllocontin 73
physical examination 36
physician's assistant 2
  see also nurse practitioner
physiotherapists 21
poison control centres 156
popliteal nerve palsy 125
postural hypotension 125, 139
posture 31, 32
Practical Diabetes 147
practice income 15
practice management 44–5
practice manager 16, 19
practice meetings 21–3
practice nurse
  activities 1–2
  as communicator 27–8
  comparison with nurse
    practitioner 3–4
  education 6–7, 143–4, 167–8
  future trends 167–8
  history 7
  professional development 1–7
  and research 6
  role 4–6, 19
    in asthma care 85–7
    in diabetes mellitus care 127, 143–4
    extended/limited 4
    in hypertension care 100–1, 107–8

Practice Receptionist Programme 19
pre-conceptual advice in diabetes
  mellitus 142
prednisolone (Prednesol) 73
pregnancy and diabetes mellitus 122
preventive medicine 24–5, 47–62
primary care facilitator
  availability 54, 55
  tasks 53
primary care team 16, 19–21
  meetings 21–3
proliferative retinopathy 124
propranolol 99
proteinuria
  in diabetes mellitus 123, 138
  in hypertension 95
psychiatric social workers 20
Pulmicort 74
pupil dilatation 140

rates, reimbursement of 15
recall systems 51–2
receptionists 19
recruitment systems 51–2
red eyes 158–61
reimbursement of direct expenses
  14, 15
relaxation classes 20
renal failure
  in diabetes mellitus 123
  and hypertension 95
renin 92
rent, reimbursement of 15
research, importance for practice
  nurses 6
respiratory tract, anatomy and
  physiology 65–7
retinopathy, diabetic 123–4
reversibility tests 70
Rotahaler 80, 81

salbutamol 72
salt
  and diabetes mellitus 145
  and hypertension 93
screening 24–5, 47–9
  protected time for 49, 51
  recruitment and recall systems
    51–2
  resources 52–3
  setting priorities 49
seizures 157–8
sensory neuropathy in diabetes
  mellitus 124
serum fructosamine 139
shared care in diabetes mellitus 127
Sikh diet in diabetes mellitus 146
skin tests in asthma 71
Slo-phyllin 73

smoking
  altering attitudes to 48
  and diabetes mellitus 116
  and hypertension 95, 98
social workers 20
sodium cromoglycate 74
spacer devices 76–80
speech, codes of 29, 30
speech therapists 21
Spinhaler 81
stress, coping with 43
stroke
  and hypertension 94
  prevention project 53–62
subarachnoid haemorrhage and
  hypertension 94
sulphonylureas 120–1
sutures 153–4
systemic steroids 73

team meetings 21–3
teamwork 21–3
  in screening clinics 62
terbutaline 72
theophylline 73
thiazide diuretics 99
Tilade 74
tolbutamide 120, 121
touching 31–2
Triflo 80
Turbohaler 80, 82

Uniphyllin 73
upper respiratory tract infection and
  asthma 67
urine testing in diabetes mellitus 134,
  138

vasoconstriction and hypertension 94
Ventide 75
Ventolin 72
verapamil 99
verbal communication 29, 30
visual acuity in diabetes mellitus 140
Volumatic 78–80
vulvitis 126

weight and hypertension 93
Working for Patients 12
wounds 152
  cleaning 152–3
  dressing 154
  instructions to patients 154–5
  suturing 153–4
Wright mini peak flow meter 71
Wycombe Primary Care Prevention
  Project 34

Zaditen 74